Assessing and Treating Anxiety Disorders in Young Children

Suneeta Monga · Diane Benoit

Assessing and Treating Anxiety Disorders in Young Children

The Taming Sneaky Fears Program

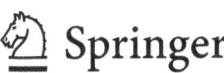 Springer

Suneeta Monga
Department of Psychiatry
Hospital for Sick Children
Toronto, ON, Canada

and

Department of Psychiatry
University of Toronto
Toronto, ON, Canada

Diane Benoit
Department of Psychiatry
Hospital for Sick Children
Toronto, ON, Canada

and

Department of Psychiatry
University of Toronto
Toronto, ON, Canada

ISBN 978-3-030-04938-6   ISBN 978-3-030-04939-3   (eBook)
https://doi.org/10.1007/978-3-030-04939-3

Library of Congress Control Number: 2018962395

This Springer imprint is published by the registered company Springer Nature Switzerland AG
The registered company address is: Gewerbestrasse 11, 6330 Cham, Switzerland

Acknowledgements

We thank the Psychiatry Endowment Fund at the Hospital for Sick Children for the early seed funding nearly two decades ago to develop the Taming Sneaky Fears program and for their financial support for the ongoing refinement of the Taming Sneaky Fears program. We are grateful to the Ontario Mental Health Foundation for funding research activities that provided the empirical evidence documenting the efficacy of the Taming Sneaky Fears program. We also thank clinicians from various community mental health agencies in Northern Ontario, Canada, with a special mention of clinicians from Algoma Family Services in Sault Ste. Marie, Ontario, who have gained an expertise in implementing the Taming Sneaky Fears program and provided us with insights on how to effectively teach this program to various professionals. We are also grateful to colleagues, trainees, parents, and children who have participated in the Taming Sneaky Fears program at the Hospital for Sick Children, Toronto, over the years for all of their invaluable feedback on the various iterations of the program.

Contents

About the Authors

Suneeta Monga, M.D., FRCPC is an Associate Professor of psychiatry at the University of Toronto. She is Medical Director of the Psychiatry Ambulatory Services and Associate Psychiatrist-in-Chief at the Hospital for Sick Children, as well as a Project Investigator in the Research Institute at the Hospital for Sick Children. Her research, educational, and clinical activities focus on the assessment and treatment of child and youth anxiety disorders with a special focus on anxiety disorders, including selective mutism, in four- to seven-year-old children and cognitive behavioral therapy as a treatment modality for anxiety and mood disorders. She has published in peer-reviewed scientific publications and has made numerous presentations on related topics across North America and abroad. She is the original developer of the Taming Sneaky Fears program and has led the empirical research of the program. She is a co-author of the children's story and companion workbook, Taming Sneaky Fears—Leo the Lion's story of bravery and Inside Leo's den: The workbook (and the French translation, *Apprivoiser les Peurs-pas-fines—L'histoire de bravoure de Léo le lionceau & Dans la tanière de Léo: le cahier de travail*).

Diane Benoit, M.D., FRCPC is a Professor of psychiatry at the University of Toronto, Project Investigator in the Research Institute at the Hospital for Sick Children, and Staff Psychiatrist at the Hospital for Sick Children in Toronto, Ontario, Canada. Her research, educational, and clinical activities focus on child–caregiver attachment relationships, the impact of violence, abuse, neglect on children, trauma-focused and attachment-focused assessments and interventions, caregivers' perceptions and subjective experience of their children and relationship with them, and the assessment and treatment of four- to seven-year-old children with anxiety disorders. She has published in peer-reviewed, scientific publications and other publications and has made numerous presentations related to these various topics across North America and abroad. She is the lead author of the children's story and companion workbook, *Taming Sneaky Fears—Leo the Lion's story of bravery and Inside Leo's den: The workbook* (and the French translation, *Apprivoiser les Peurs-pas-fines—L'histoire de bravoure de Léo le lionceau & Dans la tanière de Léo: le cahier de travail*).

Chapter 1
Anxiety Disorders in Young Children

1.1 Anxiety Versus Anxiety Disorder

Anxiety is an emotion experienced by adults and children of all ages. From an evolutionary viewpoint, anxiety played a protective role in that it forewarned threat, readied our ancestors to 'fight or flight' predators, and thus, increased the odds of survival. The 'fight or flight' response is activated when one faces a physical threat and chemicals such as adrenaline, noradrenaline, and cortisol are released into the bloodstream. These chemicals increase arousal and awareness, increase respiration and heart rates, and divert blood away from the internal organs such as the digestive tract into muscles in order to prepare the body to either 'fight' the threat, such as a predator, or to 'flight' and run as fast as one can away from the predator. Nowadays, most humans no longer face physical threats so extreme that they need to fight or flee from predators. However, the body continues to activate the 'fight or flight' response in response to present day threats, either real or perceived. For example, anxiety forewarns of present day 'threats' and might trigger the physiological 'fight or flight' response, expressed by vigilance for an approaching vehicle when crossing a street or studying hard for an impending exam. As such, anxiety and the associated 'fight or flight' response continue to benefit humans. Experiencing anxiety thus remains normative as long as it does not interfere with the day-to-day functioning of adults and children.

From a developmental viewpoint, four- to seven-year-old children experience many age-appropriate, normative fears, such as fears of the dark, monsters, and being away from caregivers. These normative fears are usually short-term, lasting a few days to a few weeks. Anxiety is normative as long as it remains circumscribed, short-term, and does not cause significant interference in functioning. An anxiety disorder can only be present when fears and worries become excessive and/or prevent children from doing age-appropriate activities such as getting to school and functioning in the school setting (e.g., speaking comfortably to teachers and peers, being dropped off without excessive distress), socializing with peers (e.g., going on play dates,

© Springer Nature Switzerland AG 2018
S. Monga and D. Benoit, *Assessing and Treating Anxiety Disorders in Young Children*, https://doi.org/10.1007/978-3-030-04939-3_1

participating in extra-curricular activities), or functioning at home (e.g., separating from parents, sleeping in their own bed).

1.2   Classification and Phenomenology

Three main classification systems can be used to diagnose anxiety disorders in young children: the Diagnostic and Statistical Manual of Mental Disorders—Fifth Edition (DSM-5; American Psychiatric Association, 2013), the International Classification of Diseases—Tenth Revision (ICD-10; World Health Organization, 2016),[1] and the Diagnostic Classification of Mental Health and Developmental Disorders of Infancy and Early Childhood (DC:0-5TM; Zero to Five, 2016). Table 1.1 provides a selected list of common anxiety diagnoses seen in young children from DSM-5, ICD-10, and DC:0-5™.

The DC:0-5™ classification system is limited to young children up to, and including age five years and has not been used extensively in published research studies pertaining to anxiety disorders in young children. Therefore, this chapter does not focus on the DC:0-5™ classification system beyond providing the aforementioned information. Given that most research studies pertaining to anxiety disorders in young children have used DSM criteria, this chapter focuses primarily on the DSM classification system (research studies that have used the ICD classification system are mentioned whenever relevant and Table 1.2 provides a comparison of symptoms between DSM-5 and ICD-10 anxiety diagnoses relevant to young children). In this chapter, we focus on the anxiety disorders that are most commonly seen in four- to seven-year-old children.

As seen in Table 1.2, all anxiety disorders seen in young children can be identified by the primary fear or worry present. With younger children, this fear or primary worry may not be clearly articulated. Therefore, parents' and/or teachers' observa-

Table 1.1 Classification of common anxiety disorders in young children (selected examples)

DSM-5	ICD-10	DC:0-5™
Separation anxiety disorder	Separation anxiety disorder of childhood	Separation anxiety disorder
Social anxiety disorder	(Social phobia) social anxiety disorder of childhood	Social anxiety disorder (social phobia)
Selective mutism	Selective mutism[a]	Selective mutism
Generalized anxiety disorder	Generalized anxiety disorder of childhood	Generalized anxiety disorder

[a] Also known as Elective mutism in ICD-10

---

[1] The World Health Organization has recently developed the Eleventh Revision (ICD-11), which was released on 18 June 2018, will be presented at the World Health Assembly in May 2019 for adoption by Member States, and will come into effect on 1 January 2022.

Table 1.2 Common anxiety disorders in four- to seven-year old children – comparison between DSM-5 and ICD-10 criteria

	DSM-5 criteria[a]	ICD-10 criteria[b]
Separation anxiety disorder (*of childhood in ICD-10*)	Developmentally inappropriate, persistent and excessive fear or anxiety around separation from major attachment figures as noted by at least three of the following: (1) distress with anticipation of or actual separation from home or major attachment figures; (2) worry about possible harm to major attachment figures (e.g., illness, injury, disasters, or death); (3) worry about experiencing an untoward event (e.g., getting lost, being kidnapped, having an accident, becoming ill); (4) reluctance or refusal to leave home, go to school or elsewhere because of fear of separation; (5) fear/reluctance about being alone or without major attachment figures; (6) reluctance or refusal to sleep away from home or to go to sleep without being near a major attachment figure; (7) nightmares about separation; (8) complaints of physical symptoms (e.g., headaches, stomachaches) when separation from major attachment figures occurs or is anticipated	At least three of the following: (1) unrealistic, persistent worry about possible harm occurring to major attachment figures or the loss of such figures; (2) unrealistic, persistent worry that some untoward event will separate child from major attachment figure; (3) persistent reluctance or refusal to go to school due to fear of separation; (4) difficulties separating at night as noted by one of: persistent reluctance or refusal to go to sleep without being near attachment figure; getting up at night to check on or sleep near attachment figure; persistent reluctance or refusal to sleep away from home; (5) persistent, inappropriate fear of being alone or without attachment figure during day; (6) nightmares about separation; (7) repeated physical symptoms upon separation; (8) excessive distress in anticipation of, during, or immediately following separation *Onset before age six* *Absence of generalized anxiety disorder of childhood*
Duration	At least four weeks	At least four weeks
Generalized anxiety disorder	Excessive anxiety and worry most days about a number of events or activities (such as school performance) with difficulty controlling the worry. At least one of the following symptoms is noted: (1) restlessness or feeling keyed up; (2) being easily fatigued; (3) irritability; (4) difficulty concentrating; (5) muscle tension; (6) sleep disturbances (e.g., difficulty falling or staying asleep)	Recurrent, excessive, intrusive anxiety or worries in at least two situations, activities, or circumstances, with at least three of the following: 1) worries about performance; (2) worries about physical health or being injured; (3) excessive worries about non-health themes; (4) free floating anxiety unrelated to specific situations; (5) frequent need for reassurance; (6) feelings of tension, inability to relax or concentrate, nervousness, difficulty falling asleep, autonomic symptoms (e.g., palpitations, sweating); (7) recurrent somatic complaints (e.g., headaches, stomachaches) *Onset in childhood or adolescence.* *Symptoms interfere on a daily basis or in a significant way in child's activities*
Duration	At least six months	At least one month

(continued)

Table 1.2 (continued)

	DSM-5 criteria[a]	ICD-10 criteria[b]
Specific phobia (*Phobic anxiety disorder of childhood in ICD-10*)	Out of proportion fear or anxiety about a specific object or situation (e.g., flying, heights, animals, receiving an injection, seeing blood). In children, crying, tantrums, freezing or clinging behavior may be noted. The object or situation almost always causes immediate fear or worry and the object or situation is actively avoided or endured with intense fear or anxiety	Persistent or recurrent fear that is developmentally appropriate but abnormal in intensity and is associated with significant social impairment *Absence of generalized anxiety disorder of childhood*
Duration	At least six months	At least four weeks
Social anxiety disorder (*of childhood in ICD-10*)	Persistent fear or worry about being observed in different social situations (e.g., having a conversation, meeting unfamiliar people), being observed (e.g., eating or drinking) and performing in front of others (e.g., giving a speech). Worry about doing something silly or embarrassing or that others will laugh at them. With children, the anxiety must be noted in peer settings and not just during interactions with adults. With children, the fear or anxiety may be noted as crying, tantrums, freezing, clinging, shrinking behaviors, or failure to speak in social situations	Persistent anxiety in social situations with unfamiliar people, including peers, as noted by socially avoidant behavior. Self-consciousness or embarrassment about appropriateness of behavior when interacting with unfamiliar people. Social interactions are restricted and significant distress and discomfort (e.g., crying, lack of spontaneous speech, or withdrawal) are noted in new or forced social situations although social relationships with familiar people are good *Abnormal degree, persistence over time, and impairment noted before the age of six.* *Absence of generalized anxiety disorder of childhood*
Duration	At least six months	At least four weeks
Selective mutism (*also known as elective mutism in ICD-10*)	Failure to speak in social situations (e.g., school) in which there is an expectation for speech despite speaking in other settings (e.g., home). Failure to speak is not due to a lack of knowledge or comfort with the language and is not better explained by a communication disorder nor does it occur exclusively during the course of autism spectrum disorder	Language expression and comprehension (assessed by individually administered standardized tests) are within two standard deviation limits for child's age. Consistent failure to speak in specific social situations (e.g., school) in which speech is expected despite speaking in other situations (e.g., home) *Absence of autism spectrum disorder, specific speech or language disorder, or lack of fluency in the expected language to be spoken*
Duration	At least one month (not limited to the first month of school)	More than four weeks

[a]One DSM-5 criterion for all disorders essentially specifies that the symptoms cannot be better explained by another medical or mental disorder; [b]One ICD-10 criterion common to all anxiety disorders specifies that the disorder does not occur as part of a broader disturbance of emotions, conduct, personality, or of a pervasive developmental disorder, psychotic disorder, or psychoactive substance use disorder

tions become important components of the diagnostic evaluation. For example, with social anxiety disorder, children may not express a fear or worry of being laughed at, although many behave in ways that suggest they do. Instead, young socially anxious children may exhibit difficult behaviors (e.g., tantrums, crying) when facing social encounters. Similarly, young children with separation anxiety may not articulate a worry about being away from their parents and instead, they may have a meltdown any time there is an impending separation. Additionally, given that some fears and worries may be normative at different developmental stages, the nature, intensity, and duration of fears and worries must be evaluated from a developmental perspective in order to determine whether they warrant a diagnosis. As such, a time period for symptom presence is specified for most diagnoses in both the DSM and ICD classification systems in order to distinguish symptoms of an anxiety disorder from normative anxiety.

1.3 Epidemiology

Anxiety disorders are among the most common psychiatric conditions (Polanczyk, Salum, Sugaya, Caye, & Rohde, 2015) with prevalence rates of between 10 and 20% reported in children and adolescents of all ages (Costello, Mustillo, Erkanli, Keeler, & Angold, 2003). Recent studies using diagnostic criteria from earlier versions of the DSM classification system (e.g., DSM-IV (American Psychiatric Association, 1994) and DSM-IV-TR (American Psychiatric Association, 2000), which are referred to as pre-DSM-5 in this chapter) and looking specifically at younger, preschool children, report prevalence rates of between 9.4 and 22%, depending upon the sample (community or pediatric primary care vs. mental health referred) and assessment method (semi-structured diagnostic interviews and parent questionnaires vs. parent questionnaires only). For example, Egger & Angold, (2006) interviewed the parents of two- to six-year-old children in a pediatric primary care setting and found that 9.4% of 307 children met criteria for an anxiety disorder based upon pre-DSM-5 criteria. By contrast, in a community sample of three-year-old children, Bufferd, Dougherty, Carlson, and Klein (2011) found that 19.6% of 541 children met criteria for at least one anxiety disorder, using pre-DSM-5 criteria. A similar prevalence rate of 19.4% was found in the Duke Preschool Anxiety Study, conducted in a pediatric primary care setting with 917 parents of two- to five-year-old children, again using pre-DSM-5 criteria (Franz, Angold, Copeland, Costello, Towe-Goodman, & Egger, 2013). Slightly higher rates of 22.2% were noted in a German sample of 1564 four- to seven-year-old children (Paulus, Backes, Sander, Weber, & von Gontard, 2014), using only a parent questionnaire based upon ICD-10 and pre-DSM-5 criteria.

Looking across the four aforementioned studies of children ranging in age from two to seven years old that used ICD-10 or pre-DSM-5 diagnostic criteria, the most common anxiety disorders in this age group appear to be separation anxiety disorder and social anxiety disorder with prevalence rates respectively ranging from 2.4 to 10.5% and 2.1 to 10.7%, followed by specific phobia with prevalence rates between

2.3 and 9%, and generalized anxiety disorder with prevalence rates ranging from 3.4 to 8.6% (Bufferd et al., 2011; Egger & Angold, 2006; Franz et al., 2013; Paulus et al., 2014).

Given that selective mutism was only placed under the umbrella of anxiety disorders in the fifth version of DSM (DSM-5) in 2013, very few studies pre-dating DSM-5 and examining the prevalence of anxiety disorders in young children have specifically examined the prevalence of selective mutism. However, as there were no major changes in the diagnostic criteria for selective mutism in DSM-5 compared to previous DSM versions, prevalence rates reported in studies looking at selective mutism using pre-DSM-5 criteria are relevant. In three studies of two- to seven-year-old children that used pre-DSM-5 diagnostic criteria, prevalence rates for selective mutism are 0.6–1.5% (Bergman, Piacentini, & McCracken, 2002; Bufferd et al., 2011; Egger & Angold, 2006).

Panic disorder, unlike the other anxiety disorders, is notably uncommon in four- to seven-year-old children. In fact, in only one study (Bufferd et al., 2011), were rates for panic disorder evaluated. Using pre-DSM-5 criteria, a 0.2% prevalence rate for panic disorder was reported in a sample of three year olds.

1.4   Comorbidity

This section examines comorbidity between the different anxiety disorders and between anxiety and non-anxiety disorders as two separate and distinct comorbidity patterns. Unfortunately, few studies have specifically examined comorbidity patterns of anxiety disorders in preschoolers so knowledge about comorbidity patterns comes indirectly from treatment studies or other types of studies, such as validation studies of diagnostic instruments. Another factor limiting current knowledge about comorbidity patterns pertains to the fact that researchers have used different diagnostic classification systems. Specifically, as seen in Table 1.2, DSM-5 and ICD-10 differ in one significant way for all anxiety disorders: ICD-10 specifically indicates that children meeting diagnostic criteria for social anxiety disorder of childhood, separation anxiety disorder of childhood, and phobic anxiety disorder of childhood cannot be diagnosed with generalized anxiety disorder of childhood; however, in DSM-5, social anxiety disorder, separation anxiety disorder, and specific phobia can all be diagnosed along with generalized anxiety disorder. This distinction was also present in earlier versions of the DSM and ICD classification systems. As a result, research studies that use the DSM diagnostic criteria are likely to document higher comorbidity amongst the various anxiety disorders given the ability to diagnose multiple anxiety disorders in the same child, whereas studies using the ICD-10 diagnostic criteria are likely to document lower comorbidity rates among anxiety disorders given the restrictions on diagnosing multiple anxiety disorders in the same child. Furthermore, to our knowledge, no study has compared comorbidity rates using both DSM and ICD diagnostic criteria in young children.

1.4.1 Comorbidity Between Anxiety Disorders

One of the few studies to look specifically at prevalence and comorbidity of anxiety disorders in preschoolers in a pediatric primary care setting, the Duke Preschool Anxiety Study ($N = 917$), examined rates of separation, social, and generalized anxiety disorders using DSM-IV-TR (American Psychiatric Association, 2000) criteria and found that 23% of two- to five-year-old children met criteria for two of the three anxiety disorders while 7% met criteria for all three anxiety disorders (Franz et al., 2013). Supporting the high comorbidity amongst the anxiety disorders in young children, a recent study of the Taming Sneaky Fears program (Monga, Rosenbloom, Tanha, Owens, & Young, 2015) found that 66 (85.7%) of 77 five- to seven-year-old children recruited to the study that took place in a tertiary care psychiatric setting had two or more DSM-IV-TR anxiety disorders and/or selective mutism, while 21 (27.3%) of 77 had three or more anxiety disorders and/or selective mutism. In other treatment studies, 77% (Hirshfeld-Becker, Masek, Henin, Blakely, Pollock-Wurman, McQuade, et al., 2010) to 87% (Waters, Ford, Wharton, & Cobham, 2009) of preschool children met DSM-IV (American Psychiatric Association, 1994) diagnostic criteria for more than one anxiety disorder.

1.4.2 Comorbidity Between Anxiety Disorders and Non-anxiety Disorders

The Duke Preschool Anxiety Study (Franz et al., 2013) is also the first study to examine the comorbidity between anxiety disorders and non-anxiety disorders in two- to five-year-old children in a pediatric primary care setting and found that 22% of children with an anxiety disorder also had oppositional defiant disorder and 17% had comorbid attention deficit hyperactivity disorder. The highest comorbidity rates of non-anxiety disorder in this study were seen in the children with generalized anxiety disorder, with 51% of them also meeting diagnostic criteria for a non-anxiety psychiatric disorder (oppositional defiant disorder or attention deficit hyperactivity disorder). Forty one percent of the children with separation anxiety disorder and 32% of children with social anxiety disorder had one of the aforementioned non-anxiety psychiatric disorders.

Lower comorbidity rates between anxiety disorders and non-anxiety disorders were reported in the Taming Sneaky Fears study (Monga et al., 2015), with 11.5% of children having both an anxiety disorder and oppositional defiant disorder and 3.9% having both an anxiety disorder and attention deficit hyperactivity disorder.

1.4.3 Comorbidity Between Selective Mutism and Social Anxiety Disorder

Approximately twenty-one studies have provided evidence for the comorbidity between selective mutism and other anxiety disorders, with 12 studies having specifically examined the co-occurrence of selective mutism and social anxiety disorder in children of all ages (see Muris & Ollendick, 2015, for a comprehensive review). Many of these studies, however, have serious methodological limitations as they are descriptive, have small sample sizes, only looked at anxiety symptoms as opposed to anxiety disorders, or only used broadband parent questionnaires such as the Child Behavior Checklist (Achenbach & Rescorla, 2001) to establish 'diagnosis.' In the context of these significant limitations, the range of co-occurrence of selective mutism and social anxiety disorder varied greatly, from a reported low of 14% of four- to 13-year-old clinically referred children with selective mutism ($N = 21$) also having social anxiety disorder in one study (Edison, Evans, McHolm, Cunningham, Nowakoswki, Bowle, & Schmidt, 2011), to 100% reported in four other studies. These latter four studies consisted of one study of 70 three- to 11-year old children with selective mutism recruited from the Web and parent oriented conferences (Chavira, Shipon-Blum, Hitchcock, Cohan, & Stein, 2007), one study of 59 three- to 17-year-old children with selective mutism recruited via advertisements and school referrals (Dummit, Klein, Tancer, Asche, Martin, & Fairbanks, 1997), one treatment study of 24 three- to nine-year-old clinically referred children with selective mutism (Oerbeck, Stein, Wentzel-Larsen, Langrud, & Kristensen, 2014), and one study of 15 four- to 19-year-old clinically referred adolescents with selective mutism (Vecchio & Kearney, 2005). These findings demonstrating the high co-occurrence of selective mutism with social anxiety disorder, especially in the younger age group, have led many clinicians and researchers to the conceptualization that the two conditions are variations of the same disorder.

1.5 Etiological Risk Factors

The available evidence suggests that biological factors such as genetics, temperament (e.g., low adaptability, high intensity of reactions), and/or behavioral inhibition, as well as environmental factors such as parental modeling, parental style, parental anxiety, and the quality of child-caregiver attachment relationship, might be involved in the etiology of anxiety disorders. Although few studies have specifically examined the development of anxiety disorders in preschool children, current evidence suggests that biological and environmental factors are likely bidirectional and their influence on the development of anxiety disorders is dependent upon other factors related to individual characteristics and family contexts.

1.5.1 *Genetics*

No genetic studies have specifically examined anxiety disorders in preschool children. The current knowledge about the familial transmission of anxiety disorders comes from studies conducted in older children and adults with anxiety disorders in which both family studies and twin studies support the familial transmission of anxiety disorders. For example, studies suggest that compared to children without an anxiety disorder, children with anxiety disorders are more likely to have a parent with an anxiety disorder (Last, Hersen, Kazdin, Francis, & Grubb, 1987; Last, Hersen, Kazdin, Orvaschel, & Perrin, 1991; Lieb, Wittchen, Hofler, Fuetsch, Stein, & Merikangas, 2000). Furthermore, a meta-analysis of family and twin studies of panic disorder, generalized anxiety disorder, phobia (including social phobia and agarophobia), and obsessive-compulsive disorder supports the familial aggregation of anxiety disorders (Hettema, Neale, & Kendler, 2001). The heritability across these various anxiety disorders, however, is modest (30–40%) and lower than that found in disorders such as schizophrenia and bipolar disorder (Hettema et al., 2001).

Several studies (Chavira et al., 2007; Kristensen & Torgersen, 2001, 2002; Remschmidt, Poller, Herpertz-Dahlmann, Henninghausen, & Gutenbrunner, 2001) demonstrate strong family histories of selective mutism or social reticence in parents and siblings of probands with selective mutism. Additionally, and in support of the genetic risk, there is early evidence to suggest that one of the polymorphisms in CNTNAP2 (*rs2710102*) is significantly associated with selective mutism (Stein, Yang, Chavira, Hitchcock, Sung, Shipon-Blum & Gelernter, 2011), as well as social anxiety symptoms and social anxiety traits.

1.5.2 *Behavioral Inhibition*

Behavioral inhibition is characterized by hypervigilance, especially in novel and unfamiliar social situations, and reticence to engage in, or withdrawal from, social interaction (e.g., looking on rather than interacting with others or playing alone) (Kagan, Reznick, & Snidman, 1987). Approximately 15–20% of normatively developing children display behavioral inhibition (Fox, Henderson, Marshall, Nichols, & Ghera, 2005), with about half of these children continuing to display this temperamental style throughout childhood (Degnan & Fox, 2007). Additionally, several longitudinal and cross-sectional studies suggest that children with behavioral inhibition are at risk for the development of anxiety disorders, especially social anxiety disorder, at a later age (e.g., Biederman, Hirshfeld-Becker, Rosenbaum, Herot, Friedman, Snidman, et al., 2001; Hayward, Killen, Kraemer, & Taylor, 1998; Schwartz, Snidman, & Kagan, 1999). However, these same studies suggest that not all children who display behavioral inhibition develop anxiety disorders as 28% of children who display behavioral inhibition do not show any diagnosable anxiety disorder, while between 39 to 83% do not meet diagnostic criteria for social anxiety disorder

(Degnan, Almas, & Fox, 2010). These findings suggest that the interplay of other factors, along with behavioral inhibition, is necessary for the development of an anxiety disorder.

Recent studies have examined more specifically the effects of behavioral inhibition in younger children. In one study, behavioral inhibition at age four years was a significant predictor of social anxiety or generalized anxiety disorder at age six years, even after controlling for baseline anxiety (Hudson, Dodd, Lyneham, & Bovopoulous, 2011). Wichstrom and colleagues (Wichstrom, Belsky, & Berg-Nielsen, 2013) used logistic regression analyses and identified the following risk factors for an anxiety disorder at age six years: high scores of behavioral inhibition, attention deficit hyperactivity disorder, parental anxiety, and peer victimization. Furthermore, poor social skills at age four were predictive of anxiety disorders at age six. Conversely, children with low behavioral inhibition at age four were protected from the effects of parental anxiety (Wichstrom et al., 2013). As such, behavioral inhibition appears to be one factor among many that contributes to the development of an anxiety disorder in young children.

1.5.3   Parenting Styles and Parental Anxiety

The role of parental anxiety in the development of anxiety disorders in children is likely due to both genetic and environmental influences. To date, the majority of studies that have examined the role of parenting styles on the development of anxiety disorders have been done in older children. In these studies, parenting that is intrusive, over-solicitous, or controlling has been associated with more social reticence and inhibition in the children (Hudson & Rapee, 2001; Rubin, Burgess, & Hastings, 2002; Rubin, Cheah, & Fox, 2001; Rubin, Hastings, Stewart, Henderson, & Chen, 1997).

More recently, studies in younger children have emerged. For example, in a study of 202 three- to four-year-old children, Hudson and colleagues (Hudson et al., 2011) found that maternal anxiety, over-involvement, negativity, and attachment were associated with children's anxiety at follow-up, but when controlling for the children's baseline anxiety, only maternal anxiety in children at age four years was a significant predictor of the children's anxiety at age six years. Additionally, in a community sample of 541 three-year-old children, those with an anxiety disorder ($N = 106$) were more likely to have a mother with a current anxiety disorder diagnosis, while there was no significant association between the children's anxiety diagnosis and an anxiety disorder in their fathers (Dougherty, Tolep, Bufferd, Olino, Dyson, Traditi, et al., 2013).

1.5.4 Additional Risk Factors Associated with Selective Mutism

Subtle language deficits and recent family migration have been hypothesized as potential factors involved in the etiology of selective mutism. For example, two studies (Manassis, Tannock, Garlan, Minde, McInnes, & Clark, 2007; McInnes, Fung, Manassis, Fiksenbaum, & Tannock, 2004) suggest that deficits in expressive and receptive language skills and in phonemic awareness on standardized language measures occur more often in children with selective mutism compared to anxious, non-selectively mute children, although not all children with selective mutism have these deficits. While three studies document an association between selective mutism and recent immigration to a new country (Dummit et al., 1997; Manassis et al., 2007; Steinhausen & Juzi, 1996), most children with selective mutism do not have a history of recent immigration to a new country.

1.6 Impact on Family Functioning

The presence of an anxiety disorder in preschool children also appears to have an impact on parental and family functioning. In an extension of the Duke Preschool Anxiety Study (Towe-Goodman, Franz, Copeland, Angold, & Egger, 2014), parents of two- to five-year-old children with an anxiety disorder completed the Child and Adolescent Impact Assessment (Angold, Patrick, Burns, & Costello, 2008) to determine the impact of young children's anxiety disorder on family functioning. Findings suggest that even after co-varying for the impact of other disorders, parents of children with an anxiety disorder were 3.5 times (OR: 95% CI = 2.4–5.3; $p < 0.0001$) more likely to report a negative impact of their children's anxiety disorder on family functioning, compared to families with same age children without an anxiety disorder. Parents across all anxiety disorders specifically reported a negative impact of their children's anxiety disorder on their own well-being, with the greatest impact reported by parents of children with generalized anxiety disorder. Parents of children with separation anxiety and generalized anxiety disorder reported a greater negative impact on their spousal relationship, which they attributed to their children's anxiety, while parents of children with social anxiety disorder reported that their children's anxiety symptoms caused them to have to restrict their own activities (e.g., social life, hobbies).

1.7 Future Directions

Despite methodological limitations of many studies reported in this chapter, current evidence suggests high prevalence rates of anxiety disorders as well as high comorbidity between the various anxiety disorders and between anxiety disorders and other non-anxiety disorders in children of all ages, including in preschool children. More research is clearly needed on the prevalence and comorbidity of anxiety disorders, specifically in young children, using the more recent DSM-5 and ICD-10 (soon to come ICD-11) diagnostic criteria, comparing the two classification systems, using larger sample sizes in both community and clinical samples, and using more stringent methodology than most studies have used to date. In addition, further exploration of the links between selective mutism and social anxiety disorder is needed, using methodologically sound approaches and universally accepted definitions and diagnostic criteria for these two disorders. Future research efforts could focus on the identification of factors involved in the development and perpetuation of anxiety disorders in young children to allow for a better conceptualization of the role, impact, and interplay of biological and developmental factors (e.g., genetic, temperament, behavioral inhibition), caregiving environment, and other environmental factors (e.g., bullying, peer victimization, family migration). The examination of the role of language deficits, family migration, and other factors in the onset and perpetuation of selective mutism in young children is also an area in need of systematic research. Finally, we welcome future research focusing on the identification of possible protective factors within the child (e.g., social competence), the caregiving environment (e.g., secure organized attachment), and/or social environment, and other moderating and mediating factors.

References

Achenbach, T. M., & Rescorla, L. A. (2001). *Manual for the ASEBA school-age forms & profiles.* Burlington, VT: University of Vermont, Research Center for Children, Youth, & Families.

American Psychiatric Association. (1994). *Diagnostic and statistical manual of mental disorders* (4th ed.) Washington, DC: American Psychiatric Association.

American Psychiatric Association. (2000). *Diagnostic and statistical manual of mental disorders* (4th ed., Text Revision). Washington, DC: American Psychiatric Association.

American Psychiatric Association. (2013). *Diagnostic and statistical manual of mental disorders* (5th ed.) Washington, DC: American Psychiatric Association.

Angold, A., Patrick, M., Burns, B. J., & Costello, E. J. (2008). *The child and adolescent impact assessment (CAIA: Version 3.0).* Durham, NC: Department of Psychiatry and Behavioral Sciences, Duke University Medical Center.

Bergman, R. L., Piacentini, J., & McCracken, J. T. (2002). Prevalence and description of selective mutism in a school-based sample. *Journal of the American Academy of Child and Adolescent Psychiatry, 41*(8), 938–946.

Biederman, J., Hirshfeld-Becker, D. R., Rosenbaum, J. F., Herot, C., Friedman, D., Snidman, N., …, Faraone, S. V. (2001). Further evidence of association between behavioral inhibition and social anxiety in children. *American Journal of Psychiatry, 158*(10), 1673–1679.

Bufferd, S. J., Dougherty, L. R., Carlson, G. A., & Klein, D. N. (2011). Parent-reported mental health in preschoolers: Findings using a diagnostic interview. *Comprehensive Psychiatry, 52,* 359–369.

Chavira, D. A., Shipon-Blum, E., Hitchcock, C., Cohan, S., & Stein, M. B. (2007). Selective mutism and social anxiety disorder: All in the family? *Journal of the American Academy of Child and Adolescent Psychiatry, 46*(11), 1464–1472.

Costello, E. J., Mustillo, S., Erkanli, A., Keeler, G., & Angold, A. (2003). Prevalence and development of psychiatric disorders in childhood and adolescence. *Archives of General Psychiatry, 60,* 837–844.

Degnan, K. A., Almas, A. N., & Fox, N. A. (2010). Temperament and the environment in the etiology of childhood anxiety. *The Journal of Child Psychology and Psychiatry, 51*(4), 497–517.

Degnan, K. A., & Fox, N. A. (2007). Behavioral inhibition and anxiety disorders: Multiple levels of a resilience process. *Development and Psychopathology, 19*(3), 729–746.

Dougherty, L. R., Tolep, M. R., Bufferd, S. J., Olino, T. M., Dyson, M., Traditi, J., …, Klein, D. N. (2013). Preschool anxiety disorders: Comprehensive assessment of clinical, demographic, temperamental, familial, and life stress correlates. *Journal of Clinical Child and Adolescent Psychology, 42*(5), 577–589.

Dummit, E. S., Klein, R. G., Tancer, N. K., Asche, B., Martin, J., & Fairbanks, J. A. (1997). Systematic assessment of 50 children with selective mutism. *Journal of the American Academy of Child and Adolescent Psychiatry, 36*(5), 653–660.

Edison, S. C., Evans, M. A., McHolm, A. E., Cunningham, C. E., Nowakoswki, M. E., Bowle, M., & Schmidt, L. A. (2011). An investigation of control among parents of selectively mute, anxious, and non-anxious children. *Child Psychiatry and Human Development, 42,* 270–290.

Egger, H. L., & Angold, A. (2006). Common emotional and behavioral disorders in preschool children: Presentation, nosology, and epidemiology. *The Journal of Child Psychology and Psychiatry, 47*(3), 313–337.

Egger, H. L., Erkanli, A., Keeler, G., Potts, E., Walter, B. K., & Angold, A. (2006). Test-retest reliability of the preschool age psychiatric assessment (PAPA). *Journal of the American Academy of Child and Adolescent Psychiatry, 45*(5), 538–549.

Fox, N. A., Henderson, H. A., Marshall, P. J., Nichols, K. E., & Ghera, M. M. (2005). Behavioral inhibition: Linking biology and behavior within a developmental framework. *Annual Review of Psychology, 56,* 235–262.

Franz, L., Angold, A., Copeland, W., Costello, E. J., Towe-Goodman, N., & Egger, H. (2013). Preschool anxiety disorders in pediatric primary care: Prevalence and comorbidity. *Journal of the American Academy of Child and Adolescent Psychiatry, 52*(12), 1294–1303.

Hayward, C., Killen, J. D., Kraemer, H. C., & Taylor, C. B. (1998). Linking self-reported childhood behavioral inhibition to adolescent social phobia. *Journal of the American Academy of Child and Adolescent Psychiatry, 37*(12), 1308–1316.

Hettema, J. M., Neale, M. C., & Kendler, K. S. (2001). A review and meta-analysis of the genetic epidemiology of anxiety disorders. *American Journal of Psychiatry, 158*(10), 1568–1578.

Hirshfeld-Becker, D. R., Masek, B., Henin, A., Blakely, L. R., Pollock-Wurman, R. A., McQuade, J., …, Biederman, J. (2010). Cognitive behavioral therapy for 4- to 7-year-old children with anxiety disorders: A randomized clinical trial. *Journal of Consulting and Clinical Psychology, 78*(4), 498–510.

Hudson, J. L., Dodd, H. F., Lyneham, H. J., & Bovopoulous, N. (2011). Temperament and family environment in the development of anxiety disorder: Two-year follow-up. *Journal of the American Academy of Child and Adolescent Psychiatry, 50*(12), 1255–1264.

Hudson, J. L., & Rapee, R. M. (2001). Parent-child interactions and anxiety disorders: An observational study. *Behaviour Research and Therapy, 39*(12), 1411–1427.

Kagan, J., Reznick, J. S., & Snidman, N. (1987). The physiology and psychology of behavioral inhibition in children. *Child Development, 58*(6), 1459–1473.

Kristensen, H., & Torgersen, S. (2001). MCMI-II personality traits and symptom traits in parents of children with selective mutism: A case-control study. *Journal of Abnormal Psychology, 110,* 648–652.

Kristensen, H., & Torgersen, S. (2002). A case-control study of EAS child and parental temperaments in selectively mute children with and without a co-morbid communication disorder. *Nordic Journal of Psychiatry, 56*(5), 347–353.

Last, C. G., Hersen, M., Kazdin, A. E., Francis, G., & Grubb, H. J. (1987). Psychiatric illness in the mothers of anxious children. *American Journal of Psychiatry, 144*(12), 1580–1583.

Last, C. G., Hersen, M., Kazdin, A. E., Orvaschel, H., & Perrin, S. (1991). Anxiety disorders in children and their families. *Archives of General Psychiatry, 48*(10), 928–934.

Lieb, M., Wittchen, H. U., Hofler, M., Fuetsch, M., Stein, M. B., & Merikangas, K. R. (2000). Parental psychopathology, parenting styles, and the risk of social phobia in offspring. *Archives of General Psychiatry, 57,* 859–866.

Manassis, K., Tannock, R., Garland, J., Minde, K., McInnes, A., & Clark, S. (2007). The sounds of silence: Language, cognition, and anxiety in selective mutism. *Journal of the American Academy of Child and Adolescent Psychiatry, 46*(9), 1187–1195.

McInnes, A., Fung, D., Manassis, K., Fiksenbaum, L., & Tannock, R. (2004). Narrative skills in children with selective mutism: An exploratory study. *American Journal of Speech-Language Pathology, 13*(4), 304–315.

Monga, S., Rosenbloom, B., Tanha, A., Owens, M., & Young, A. (2015). Comparison of child-parent and parent-only cognitive-behavioral therapy programs for anxious Children aged 5 to 7 years: Short- and long-term outcomes. *Journal of the American Academy of Child and Adolescent Psychiatry, 54*(2), 138–146.

Muris, P., & Ollendick, T. H. (2015). Children who are anxious in silence: A review on selective mutism, the new anxiety disorder in DSM-5. *Clinical Child and Family Psychology Review, 18,* 151–169.

Oerbeck, B., Stein, M. B., Wentzel-Larsen, T., Langrud, O., & Kristensen, H. (2014). A randomized controlled trial of a home and school-based intervention for selective mutism: Defocused communication and behavioral techniques. *Child and Adolescent Mental Health, 19,* 192–198.

Paulus, F. W., Backes, A., Sander, C. S., Weber, M., & von Gontard, A. (2014). Anxiety disorders and behavioral inhibition in preschool children: A population-based study. *Child Psychiatry and Human Development, 46*(1), 150–157.

Polanczyk, G. V., Salum, G. A., Sugaya, L. S., Caye, A., & Rohde, L. A. (2015). Annual research review: A meta-analysis of the worldwide prevalence of mental disorders in children and adolescents. *Journal of Child Psychology and Psychiatry, 56*(3), 345–365.

Remschmidt, H., Poller, M., Herpertz-Dahlmann, B., Henninghausen, K., & Gutenbrunner, C. (2001). A follow-up study of 45 patients with elective mutism. *European Archives of Psychiatry and Clinical Neuroscience, 251*(6), 284–296.

Rubin, K. H., Burgess, K. B., & Hastings, P. S. (2002). Stability and social-behavioral consequences of toddlers' inhibited temperament and parenting behaviors. *Child Development, 73*(2), 483–495.

Rubin, K. H., Cheah, C. S. L., & Fox, N. (2001). Emotional regulation, parenting and display of social reticence in preschoolers. *Early Education and Development, 12*(1), 97–115.

Rubin, K. H., Hastings, P. D., Stewart, S. L., Henderson, H. A., & Chen, X. (1997). The consistency and concomitants of inhibition: Some of the children, all of the time. *Child Development, 68,* 467–483.

Schwartz, C. E., Snidman, N., & Kagan, J. (1999). Adolescent social anxiety as an outcome of inhibited temperament in childhood. *Journal of the American Academy of Child and Adolescent Psychiatry, 38*(8), 1008–1015.

Stein, M. B., Yang, B. Z., Chavira, D. A., Hitchcock, C. A., Sung, S. C., Shipon-Blum, E., & Gelernter, J. (2011). A common genetic variant in the neurexin superfamily member CNTNAP2 is associated with increased risk for selective mutism and social anxiety-related traits. *Biological Psychiatry, 69*(9), 825–831.

Steinhausen, H.-C., & Juzi, C. (1996). Elective mutism: An analysis of 100 causes. *Journal of the American Academy of Child and Adolescent Psychiatry, 35*(5), 606–614.

Towe-Goodman, N. R., Franz, L., Copeland, W., Angold, A., & Egger, H. (2014). Perceived family impact of preschool anxiety disorders. *Journal of the American Academy of Child and Adolescent Psychiatry, 53*(4), 437–446. https://doi.org/10.1016/j.jaac.2013.12.017.

Vecchio, J. L., & Kearney, C. A. (2005). Selective mutism in children: Comparison to youths with and without anxiety disorders. *Journal of Psychopathology and Behavioral Assessment, 27,* 31–37.

Waters, A. M., Ford, L. A., Wharton, T. A., & Cobham, V. E. (2009). Cognitive-behavioural therapy for young children with anxiety disorders: Comparison of a Child + Parent condition versus a Parent Only condition. *Behaviour Research and Therapy, 47*(8), 654–662.

Wichstrom, L., Belsky, J., & Berg-Nielsen, T. S. (2013). Preschool predictors of childhood anxiety disorders: A prospective community study. *Journal of Child Psychology and Psychiatry, 54*(12), 1327–1336.

World Health Organization (2016). *International statistical classification of diseases and related health problems*, 10th Revision (10 ed.). Geneva: World Health Organization.

Zero to Five. (2016). *Diagnostic classification of mental health and developmental disorders of infancy and early childhood*. Washington, DC: Zero to Five Press.

Chapter 2
Screening and Assessment Tools for Young Anxious Children

2.1 Anxiety-Specific Screening Tools for Four-to Seven-Year-Old Children

The paucity of methodologically sound research studies pertaining to young anxious children that was highlighted in Chap. 1, is again evident when examining screening and assessment tools for anxiety symptoms in four- to seven-year-old children. With only a few instruments having been specifically developed to screen and assess anxiety symptoms in four- to seven-year-old children, the field is characterized by a dearth of universally accepted and validated screening and assessment tools for this age group. Further, as described below, some of these instruments have not been thoroughly validated in young children and somewhat limited information about their psychometric properties is available, suggesting that they be used with caution in clinical settings. Nonetheless, they are described as they are currently used in clinical and research settings and some show promise.

2.1.1 Preschool Anxiety Scale

The Preschool Anxiety Scale (Spence & Rapee, 1999) consists of a 29-item parent questionnaire and a 22-item teacher questionnaire for use with three- to six-year-old children. Several questionnaire items were taken from the Spence Children's Anxiety Scale (Spence, 1997; Spence, 1998), a tool for use with older children, and reworded for use with the parents of preschool children. The parent and teacher versions of the Preschool Anxiety Scale are described in more detail below (Sects. 2.1.1.1 and 2.1.1.2).

© Springer Nature Switzerland AG 2018
S. Monga and D. Benoit, *Assessing and Treating Anxiety Disorders in Young Children*, https://doi.org/10.1007/978-3-030-04939-3_2

2.1.1.1 Preschool Anxiety Scale—Parent Questionnaire

In the Preschool Anxiety Scale—Parent Questionnaire, parents report on their three-to six-year-old children's anxiety symptoms in different scenarios (e.g., when swimming, facing heights, with insects, in the classroom) using a 5-point Likert-type scale with $0 = $ not true at all, $1 = $ seldom true, $2 = $ sometimes true, $3 = $ quite often true, and $4 = $ very often true. If children have experienced a traumatic event, parents complete an additional five items.

The psychometric properties of the Preschool Anxiety Scale–Parent Questionnaire were examined in a sample of 755 mothers of preschool and kindergarten-aged children between the ages of 31–83 months (Spence, Rapee, McDonald, & Ingram, 2001). Confirmatory factor analysis identified five factors that make up the five subscales of the instrument (social anxiety, separation anxiety, obsessive-compulsive symptoms, fear of physical injury, and generalized anxiety). The sum of the five subscale scores yields a total score. A subsample of 472 mothers completed both the Preschool Anxiety Scale—Parent Questionnaire and the Child Behavior Checklist (Achenbach & Rescorla, 2001), a broadband measure of internalizing and externalizing problems in children. Convergent validity was established by comparing the total score of the Preschool Anxiety Scale—Parent Questionnaire and the internalizing subscale of the Child Behavior Checklist, $r = 0.68$ ($p < 0.001$). Additionally, each of the five Preschool Anxiety Scale—Parent Questionnaire subscales individually correlated positively with the Child Behavior Checklist internalizing subscale (p values were not reported), including generalized anxiety, $r = 0.60$; social anxiety, $r = 0.57$; separation anxiety, $r = 0.50$; obsessive-compulsive symptoms, $r = 0.42$; and fear of physical injury, $r = 0.43$. Lower, although still significant correlations ($r = 0.21$, $p < 0.001$), were noted between mothers' total scores on the Preschool Anxiety Scale—Parent Questionnaire and mothers' scores on the broadband externalizing subscale of the Child Behavior Checklist (Spence et al., 2001).

The Preschool Anxiety Scale—Parent Questionnaire is the most commonly used anxiety-specific screening tool for children under the age of eight years, and to date, it is the best-studied instrument of its kind in this young age group. Further validation of the Preschool Anxiety Scale—Parent Questionnaire would provide greater evidence to support its use in clinical and research settings.

2.1.1.2 Preschool Anxiety Scale—Teacher Questionnaire

The Preschool Anxiety Scale—Teacher Questionnaire (Spence & Rapee, 1999) is a 22-item questionnaire for use by teachers of children three to six years of age. Teachers rate items describing children's anxiety in various school-related situations, using the same 5-point Likert-type scale as the Preschool Anxiety Scale—Parent Questionnaire. The Preschool Anxiety Scale—Teacher Questionnaire yields the same five subscales as the Preschool Anxiety Scale—Parent Questionnaire: social anxiety, separation anxiety, obsessive-compulsive symptoms, fears of physical injury, and generalized anxiety. No psychometric data are available on the Preschool Anxiety Scale—Teacher Questionnaire and currently this tool is restricted to research studies in which norms are not required.

2.1.2 Picture Anxiety Test

The Picture Anxiety Test (Dubi & Schneider, 2009) is a clinician-administered instrument to assess anxiety and avoidance in four- to eight-year-old children. Developed originally in the German language, an English translation is also available. The Picture Anxiety Test uses color pictures rather than text to engage and encourage participation of young children. Seventeen items make up the full test: 11 for specific phobia, two for social anxiety, two for generalized anxiety, and two for separation anxiety. For each item, two color illustrations of children of the same gender as the child being assessed are presented simultaneously: the child in one illustration is responding in an anxious or fearful manner while the child in the other illustration is responding in a neutral manner. The test consists of having the clinician ask the child to choose the picture that best resembles the child's own reaction to the illustrated scenario and then ask the child to use a four-point scale (ranging from $0 =$ not at all to $3 =$ very much) to rate how anxious the child would feel if faced with the illustrated situation. Using the same four-point scale, the clinician also asks how much the child would avoid the illustrated situation. Clinical judgment may be used to adjust the ratings provided by the child. The Picture Anxiety Test yields three scores: an anxiety score encapsulating the ratings of how anxious the child would feel in a given situation, an avoidance score derived from the ratings as to how much the child would avoid the situation, and a composite score determined by the sum of the anxiety score with the avoidance score.

Using a sample of 71 five- to seven-year-old children, internal consistency was established at $\alpha = 0.73$ for the anxiety score and $\alpha = 0.74$ for the avoidance score on the Picture Anxiety Test (Dubi & Schneider, 2009). Test-retest stability (over four to six weeks) was assessed in a subsample ($N = 22$) and yielded the following results: for the composite score, $r = 0.49$, $p < 0.05$; anxiety score, $r = 0.63$, $p < 0.01$; and avoidance score, $r = 0.30$, $p =$ n.s. (Dubi & Schneider, 2009).

To assess convergent validity, the questions from the Revised Children's Manifest Anxiety Scale (Reynolds & Richmond, 1978; German version: Boehnke, Silbereisen, Reynolds, & Richmond, 1986), an instrument designed for use with six- to nine-year-old anxious children, were read to the children by a clinician. Significant correlations were found between the children's scores on the Revised Children's Manifest Anxiety Scale and the Picture Anxiety Test anxiety score ($r = 0.47$, $p < 0.001$), avoidance score ($r = 0.41$, $p < 0.01$) and composite score ($r = 0.45$, $p < 0.001$). Parents also completed the parent version of the Revised Children's Manifest Anxiety Scale

(Pina, Silverman, Saavedra, & Weems, 2001; German version: Schneider, Adornetto, & Blatter, 2004) and correlations between mothers' scores on this parent instrument and the children's Picture Anxiety Test scores in general were lower: anxiety score, $r = 0.31$, $p < 0.01$; avoidance score, $r = 0.24$, $p =$ n.s.; and composite score, $r = 0.28$, $p < 0.05$ (Dubi & Schneider, 2009).

Additionally, parents completed the Child Behavior Checklist (Achenbach, 1991; German version: Döpfner, Melchers, Fegert, Lehmkuhl, Lehmkuhl, & Schmeck, et al., 1993). Significant correlations between mothers' scores on the internalizing subscale of the Child Behavior Checklist and children's scores on the Picture Anxiety Test anxiety score ($r = 0.27$, $p < 0.05$), avoidance score ($r = 0.22$, $p =$ n.s.) and composite score ($r = 0.29$, $p < 0.05$) suggest convergent validity while discriminant validity was suggested by non-significant correlations (r values $= 0.14$ to 0.22; $p =$ n.s.) between children's scores on the Picture Anxiety Test and mothers' scores on the externalizing subscale of the Child Behavior Checklist (Dubi & Schneider, 2009).

Although the use of illustrations has appeal in the under eight years age group, the Picture Anxiety Test has limitations as, for example, it requires clinician administration and focuses primarily on specific phobias rather than other anxiety symptoms.

2.2 Questionnaires Specific to Selective Mutism

Only two instruments are currently available to screen and/or assess selective mutism symptoms in four- to seven-year-old children. These include the Selective Mutism Questionnaire (Bergman, Keller, Piacentini, & Bergman, 2008) and the School Speech Questionnaire (Bergman, Keller, Wood, Piacentini, & McCracken, 2001). As with the aforementioned instruments, these questionnaires have undergone somewhat limited psychometric testing and have been used with children of a wide age range. However, despite these limitations, and perhaps because of the paucity of instruments focusing on selective mutism, the Selective Mutism Questionnaire has been used in most research studies pertaining to selective mutism and so it is described in more detail below. The School Speech Questionnaire is also discussed in more detail below.

2.2.1 Selective Mutism Questionnaire

The Selective Mutism Questionnaire (Bergman et al., 2008) is a 17-item parent questionnaire that assesses the degree and frequency of speech in three- to 11-year-old children and provides a proxy measure of selective mutism severity. Parents report on their children's behavior with regards to speaking in the previous two weeks across three broad domains (or subscales): at school (five items), at home/with family (five items), and in social situations (seven items). Parents rate items using a three-point scale that ranges from 0 = never to 3 = always. Items are summed to create a total score, with lower total scores suggesting less speech. Six additional items assess the degree of overall interference or distress experienced, although these items are not included in the total score and are used primarily for qualitative purposes.

The psychometric properties of the Selective Mutism Questionnaire were examined in studies of parents of children with or without selective mutism who attended an anxiety clinic (Bergman et al., 2008). The selective mutism group was made up of 48 children (M age $= 5.83$ years; $SD = 1.65$; range $= 3–10$) with a primary DSM-IV (American Psychiatric Association, 1994) diagnosis of selective mutism and 92% having a comorbid DSM-IV (American Psychiatric Association, 1994) social anxiety disorder diagnosis. The non-selective mutism group was made up of 18 children (M age $= 6.33$ years; $SD = 1.78$; range $= 3–10$) with a non-selective mutism anxiety disorder such as obsessive-compulsive disorder, separation anxiety disorder, generalized anxiety disorder, specific phobia, and included three children with social anxiety disorder. In the selective mutism group, internal consistency of the Selective Mutism Questionnaire was $\alpha = 0.97$ for the total score, $\alpha = 0.97$ for the school subscale, $\alpha = 0.88$ for the home/family subscale, and $\alpha = 0.96$ for the social subscale. Additionally, children in the selective mutism group were noted to have significantly less speech (M total score $= 12.99$; $SD = 7.23$) than children in the non-selective mutism group (M total score $= 46.00$; $SD = 5.94$), $t(64) = 16.05$, $p < 0.001$.

As seen in Table 2.1, to examine convergent validity, Bergman and colleagues (Bergman et al., 2008) compared the total score and subscale scores of the Selective Mutism Questionnaire with various measures of social anxiety that have been used with older children, including the parent report of the Social Anxiety Scale for Children—Revised (La Greca & Stone, 1993), an instrument validated for children in grades four to six, the parent version of the Multidimensional Anxiety Scale for Children (March, Parker, Sullivan, Stallings, & Conners, 1997), an anxiety screen validated for children eight years and older, and the Clinician Severity Rating of the clinician-administered Anxiety Disorders Interview Schedule (Silverman & Albano, 1996).

As noted in Table 2.1, Bergman and colleagues (Bergman et al., 2008) reported significant correlations between the total score on the Selective Mutism Questionnaire and (1) the social anxiety subscale score of the parent Multidimensional Anxiety Scale for Children (March et al., 1997), (2) the Clinician Severity Rating on the Anxiety Disorders Interview Schedule (Silverman & Albano, 1996), and (3) the total score of the Social Anxiety Scale for Children—Revised (La Greca & Stone, 1993). Further, when five items related to talking from the Social Anxiety Scale for Children—Revised (La Greca & Stone, 1993) were removed, the total score of the Selective Mutism Questionnaire continued to correlate significantly with the score on the remaining items. These findings provide some evidence for the convergent validity of the Selective Mutism Questionnaire with other measures assessing similar and/or related concepts, such as social anxiety symptoms.

Table 2.1 Correlations between Selective Mutism Questionnaire Total Score and other Measures

Measure	Selective Mutism Questionnaire Total Score r (p value)
Parent MASC social anxiety subscale	−0.62 (<0.01)
ADIS Clinician Severity Rating	−0.67 (<0.001)
SASC-R total score	−0.52 (<0.01)
SASC-R without talking items	−0.44 (<0.05)
Parent MASC harm avoidance subscale	0.32 (n.s.)
Parent MASC separation anxiety subscale	0.17 (n.s.)
Parent MASC physical symptoms subscale	−0.15 (n.s.)
Parent MASC total score	−0.21 (n.s.)

SASC-R Social Anxiety Scale for Children—Revised; *MASC* Multidimensional Scale for Children; *ADIS* Anxiety Disorders Interview Schedule

Conversely, as noted in Table 2.1, non-significant correlations between the total score of the Selective Mutism Questionnaire and non-social anxiety measures such as the other subscales of the parent version of the Multidimensional Anxiety Scale for Children (March et al., 1997) were observed, thus providing some evidence for discriminant validity of the Selective Mutism Questionnaire.

To assess for sensitivity to treatment response, the Selective Mutism Questionnaire was completed pre- and post-treatment in a small subsample ($N = 11$) of children with selective mutism who participated in a behavioral treatment program (Bergman et al., 2008). Paired t-tests demonstrated that the mean total Selective Mutism Questionnaire scores increased significantly from pre-treatment to post-treatment ($M = 13.83$, $SD = 5.00$ vs. $M = 31.07$, $SD = 7.01$; $p < 0.001$), indicating a significant increase in speaking behaviors post-treatment and demonstrating that the Selective Mutism Questionnaire can be used to detect change in treatment studies. Other treatment studies (e.g., Bergman, Gonzalez, Piacentini, & Keller, 2013; Sharkey, McNicholas, Barry, Begley, & Ahern, 2008) also suggest that the Selective Mutism Questionnaire can detect change in speaking behavior as a result of treatment.

The Selective Mutism Questionnaire is currently the only questionnaire that evaluates speaking behaviors in a broad age range of children and to date it has been used by most researchers as a proxy measure of symptom severity in selective mutism. Significant correlations between the Selective Mutism Questionnaire and measures of social anxiety, as described herein, suggest that the Selective Mutism Questionnaire is measuring a similar construct. The lack of a significant correlation between the Selective Mutism Questionnaire and anxiety symptoms other than social anxiety, suggests that the Selective Mutism Questionnaire is not measuring these non-social anxiety symptoms. Further research pertaining to the development and validation of screening tools that specifically evaluate the symptoms of selective mutism in four- to seven-year-old children, beyond not speaking, is warranted.

2.2.2 School Speech Questionnaire

The School Speech Questionnaire (Bergman et al., 2001) is an adaptation of the Selective Mutism Questionnaire for use with teachers of children aged three to 11 years. Teachers report on children's speaking behavior and frequency in the school setting in the previous month using the same three-point scale that is used in the Selective Mutism Questionnaire, such that lower scores reflect fewer speaking behaviors. It has undergone several revisions over the years and currently (Bergman et al., 2013), the School Speech Questionnaire is a six-item questionnaire for teachers who rate children's speaking behaviors at school on a four-point scale ranging from 0 = never to 3 = always. Lower scores indicate greater severity of impairment. In the latest treatment study conducted by the developer of the School Speech Questionnaire, internal consistency was reported as $\alpha = 0.76$ (Bergman et al., 2013).

The School Speech Questionnaire is the only currently available instrument for teachers to assess for symptoms of selective mutism in young children in the school setting. However, there is a paucity of data to document its construct validity, test-retest reliability, and other psychometric properties. The development of additional screening and assessment tools for selective mutism within the school setting is warranted.

2.3 Diagnostic Assessment Tools for Young Anxious Children

The use of validated, structured, or semi-structured interviews in research studies ensures that psychiatric diagnoses are established in a consistent and structured manner in all subjects. Two diagnostic interviews used to assess anxiety disorders in preschool children are the Anxiety Disorders Interview Schedule for DSM-IV (Silverman & Albano, 1996) and the Preschool Age Psychiatric Assessment (Egger, Ascher, & Angold, 1999). Although the validity and other psychometric properties of the Anxiety Disorders Interview Schedule for DSM-IV have been established on children older than four to seven years old, this instrument is described in more detail below because it is the instrument that is the most often used in studies of younger anxious children.

2.3.1 Anxiety Disorders Interview Schedule for DSM-IV

The Anxiety Disorders Interview Schedule for DSM-IV (ADIS; Silverman & Albano, 1996) is a semi-structured, clinician-administered, interview of parents (ADIS-P) or interview of children (ADIS-C) designed specifically to diagnose anxiety and other related disorders in children and adolescents. In addition to all of the childhood anxiety disorders, the ADIS assesses for nine other childhood disorders (e.g., mood disorder, oppositional defiant disorder, conduct disorder, attention deficit hyperactivity disorder, enuresis, obsessive-compulsive disorder). Along with symptom endorsement, children and parents are asked to rate for interference or impairment using a 9-point scale ranging from 0 to 8, with 0 being no impairment or no interference and 8 being significant impairment or interference. Additionally, the clinician conducting the interview generates an overall Clinician Severity Rating of impairment. A Clinician Severity Rating of 4 (moderate degree of impairment) or greater is required to establish presence of a diagnosis.

To examine the psychometric characteristics of the ADIS, one assessor interviewed 62 seven- to 16-year-old children (M age $= 10.15$ years) and their parents individually on two different occasions, seven to 14 days apart (Silverman, Saavedra, & Pina, 2001). After each interview, the assessor determined DSM-IV (American Psychiatric Association, 1994) diagnoses based upon the child interview alone, the parent interview alone, and the two separate interviews considered together. Data were reported for an older age group (12- to 16-year-old children; $N = 23$) and for a younger age group (7- to 11-year-old children; $N = 39$); however only data for the younger age group are reported below.

Kappa coefficients were used to examine the agreement between a specific anxiety disorder diagnosis and specific anxiety symptoms, using Landis and Koch's (1977) criteria of $\kappa > 0.81$ signifying almost perfect agreement between categorical variables, $\kappa = 0.61$ to 0.80 representing substantial agreement, $\kappa = 0.41$ to 0.60 demonstrating moderate agreement, and $\kappa = 0.21$ to 0.40 meaning fair agreement. Using the child interview alone (ADIS-C) the κ coefficients for separation anxiety disorder, social phobia, specific phobia, and generalized anxiety disorder ranged from 0.71 to 0.84, demonstrating substantial to almost perfect agreement. Similarly, using the parent interview alone (ADIS-P), the κ coefficients reflected substantial to almost perfect agreement, with κ coefficients for each of the aforementioned anxiety diagnoses ranging from 0.73 to 0.92. When both child and parent interviews (ADIS-C and ADIS-P) were used together to establish diagnosis in the younger children, the κ coefficients demonstrated almost perfect agreement, with all κ coefficients $= 0.84$ or 0.85. Intraclass correlations were used to assess reliability of symptom scale scores and ranged from 0.86 to 0.99 for parent interview, while intraclass correlations for child interview ranged from 0.85 to 0.92. Additionally, to assess for consistency in Clinician Severity Rating of impairment over time, Pearson correlations were conducted at two time points (M interval $= 11.7$ days; range 7–14) and were $r = 0.8$ for separation anxiety, $r = 0.84$ for social anxiety, $r = 0.84$ for specific phobia, and $r = 0.82$ for generalized anxiety (no p values were reported; Silverman et al., 2001).

The Anxiety Disorders Interview Schedule is currently the most commonly used diagnostic interview in treatment outcome studies for anxiety disorders in older children and adolescents (Schniering, Hudson, & Rapee, 2000). Further, even in the burgeoning field of treatment studies in younger children, the ADIS-P has been widely used to establish anxiety disorder diagnoses (e.g., Bergman et al., 2013;

Comer et al., 2012; Monga, Rosenbloom, Tanha, Owens, & Young, 2015; Monga, Young, & Owens, 2009; Oerbeck, Stein, Pripp, & Kristensen, 2015; Pincus, Santucci, Ehrenreich, & Eyberg, 2008; Waters, Ford, Wharton, & Cobham, 2009).

2.3.2 Preschool Age Psychiatric Assessment

The Preschool Age Psychiatric Assessment (Egger et al., 1999) is a structured parent interview developed to assess DSM-IV-TR (American Psychiatric Association, 2000) disorders in children aged two to five years. It was adapted from the parent version of the Child and Adolescent Psychiatric Assessment (Angold, Prendergast, Cox, Harrington, Simonoff, & Rutter, 1995), a reliable and valid measure of psychopathology in children aged nine to 18 years. The Preschool Age Psychiatric Assessment assesses for anxiety disorder, mood disorder, oppositional defiant disorder, conduct disorder, attention deficit hyperactivity disorder, as well as enuresis and encopresis based on DSM-IV-TR criteria. It contains 25 modules, which can be administered separately or in any combination, assesses disturbance in 30 areas including, for example, the child's relationship with his or her parents, and others, or the child's functioning in the home, at school, or elsewhere.

Egger, Erkanli, Keeler, Potts, Walter, & Angold (2006) examined the psychometric properties of the Preschool Age Psychiatric Assessment with 1073 parents of two- to five-year-old children who were attending a pediatric clinic. The parents completed the Child Behavior Checklist/1½–5 (Achenbach & Rescorla, 2001) and an initial diagnostic interview using the Preschool Age Psychiatric Assessment. A second interview was conducted about one week later (M interval $= 11$ days; range $=$ three days to one month) by a different clinician who was blind to the results of the first interview. Kappa coefficients were used to assess agreement on categorical variables between the two time points. Kappa coefficients for the various anxiety disorders were as follows: $\kappa = 0.36$ for specific phobia, $\kappa = 0.39$ for generalized anxiety, $\kappa = 0.53$ for selective mutism, $\kappa = 0.54$ for social anxiety, $\kappa = 0.60$ for separation anxiety disorder, and $\kappa = 0.49$ for any anxiety disorder. These κ coefficients, using Landis and Koch's (1977) criteria as described above, demonstrate fair to moderate reliability. Kappa coefficients for non-anxiety disorders were generally higher and in the moderate to substantial agreement range, i.e., depression ($\kappa = 0.72$), attention deficit hyperactivity disorder ($\kappa = 0.74$), oppositional defiant disorder ($\kappa = 0.57$), and conduct disorder ($\kappa = 0.60$). Intraclass correlations were used to assess agreement between syndrome scale scores and ranged from a low of 0.57 for specific phobia to a high of 0.73 for social anxiety disorder, with intraclass correlation $= 0.74$ for any anxiety disorder. Again, higher intraclass correlations were generally noted for the behavioral disorders and depression, with a low of 0.67 for oppositional defiant disorder to 0.80 for attention deficit hyperactivity disorder (see Egger et al., 2006, for more details).

Although the Preschool Age Psychiatric Assessment is a semi-structured interview developed specifically to assess psychiatric disorders in two- to five-year-old children, to date it has not been used extensively in studies evaluating treatment of preschool anxiety disorders.

2.4 Summary

In summary, only a few instruments, with generally limited evidence pertaining to their psychometric properties, are currently available to specifically screen for anxiety symptoms and assess anxiety disorders in four- to seven-year-old children. As described within this chapter, many of the current screening and assessment tools for young children are derived from screening tools used with older children and use symptoms and terminology that might not be particularly well suited for young children. Further, many currently available screening tools were validated against the internalizing subscale of the Child Behavior Checklist (Achenbach & Rescorla, 2001). This subscale, however, is a broadband measure of internalizing symptoms, which includes anxiety but also includes a number of mood and emotional regulation symptoms. Given the increased recognition of the high prevalence of anxiety disorders in young children (described in Chap. 1) and the paucity of validated and user-friendly assessment tools, more research is needed. We welcome future research that uses stringent designs and methods to develop and validate screening and assessment tools specifically for anxious four- to seven-year-old children that takes into consideration the unique developmental needs and cognitive abilities of young children as well as their parents' ability to recognize and report on the signs and symptoms of anxiety in their young children. In Chap. 3, we discuss some of the current tools our group is developing in an attempt to improve the screening and assessment of young children with anxiety disorders, with a specific emphasis on selective mutism and social anxiety disorder.

References

Achenbach, T. M., & Rescorla, L. A. (2001). *Manual for the ASEBA school-age forms & profiles.* Burlington, VT: University of Vermont, Research Center for Children, Youth, & Families.

Achenbach, T. M. (1991). *Manual for the child behavior checklist/4-18 and 1991 profile.* Burlington, VT: University of Vermont, Department of Psychiatry.

American Psychiatric Association. (1994). *Diagnostic and statistical manual of mental disorders* (4th ed.). Washington, DC: American Psychiatric Association.

American Psychiatric Association. (2000). *Diagnostic and statistical manual of mental disorders* (4th ed., Text Revision). Washington, DC: American Psychiatric Association.

Angold, A., Prendergast, M., Cox, A., Harrington, R., Simonoff, E., & Rutter, M. (1995). The Child and Adolescent Psychiatric Assessment (CAPA). *Psychological Medicine, 25,* 739–753.

Bergman, R. L., Gonzalez, A., Piacentini, J., & Keller, M. L. (2013). Integrated behavior therapy for selective mutism: A randomized controlled pilot study. *Behavior Research and Therapy, 51*(10), 680–689. https://doi.org/10.1016/j.brat.2013.07.003.

Bergman, R. L., Keller, M. L., Piacentini, J., & Bergman, A. J. (2008). The development and psychometric properties of the selective mutism questionnaire. *Journal of Clinical Child and Adolescent Psychology, 37*(2), 456–464.

Bergman, R. L., Keller, M., Wood, J., Piacentini, J., & McCracken, J. (2001). Selective mutism questionnaire: Development and findings. *Proceedings of the American Academy of Child and Adolescent Psychiatry Meeting, 48*, 163.

Boehnke, K., Silbereisen, R. K., Reynolds, C. R., & Richmond, B. O. (1986). What I think and feel: German experience with the revised form of the children's manifest anxiety scale. *Personality and Individual Differences, 7*(4), 553–560.

Comer, J. S., Puliafico, A. C., Aschenbrand, S. G., McKnight, K., Robin, J. A., Goldfine, M. E., & Albano, A. M. (2012). A pilot feasibility evaluation of the CALM Program for anxiety disorders in early childhood. *Journal of Anxiety Disorders, 26*(1), 40–49. https://doi.org/10.1016/j.janxdis.2011.08.011.

Döpfner, M., Melchers, P., Fegert, J., Lehmkuhl, G., Lehmkuhl, U., & Schmeck, K., et. al., (1993). Deutschsprachige Konsensus Versionen der Child Behavior Checklist (CBCL 4-18), der Teacher Report Form (TRF) und der Youth Self Report Form (YSR). *Kindheit und Entwicklung, 3*, 54–59.

Dubi, K., & Schneider, S. (2009). The picture anxiety test (PAT): A new pictorial assessment of anxiety symptoms in young children. *Journal of Anxiety Disorders, 23*, 1148–1157.

Egger, H. L., Ascher, B. H., & Angold, A. (1999). *The preschool age psychiatric assessment: Version 1. 1. unpublished interview schedule.* Durham, NC: Centre for Developmental Epidemiology, Department of Psychiatry and Behavioral Sciences, Duke University Medical Center.

Egger, H. L., Erkanli, A., Keeler, G., Potts, E., Walter, B. K., & Angold, A. (2006). Test-retest reliability of the preschool age psychiatric assessment (PAPA). *Journal of the American Academy of Child and Adolescent Psychiatry, 45*(5), 538–549.

La Greca, A. M., & Stone, W. L. (1993). The social anxiety scale for children—Revised: Factor structure and concurrent validity. *Journal of Clinical Child Psychology, 22*, 17–27.

Landis, J. R., & Koch, G. G. (1977). The Measurement of observer agreement for categorical data. *Biometric, 33*, 159–174. http://dx.doi.org/10.2307/2529310

March, J. S., Parker, J. D., Sullivan, K., Stallings, P., & Conners, C. K. (1997). The multidimensional anxiety scale for children (MASC): Factor structure, reliability, and validity. *Journal of the American Academy of Child and Adolescent Psychiatry, 36*(4), 554–565. https://doi.org/10.1097/00004583-199704000-00019.

Monga, S., Rosenbloom, B. N., Tanha, A., Owens, M., & Young, A. (2015). Comparison of child-parent and parent-only cognitive-behavioral therapy programs for anxious children aged 5 to 7 years: Short- and long-term outcomes. *Journal of the American Academy of Child and Adolescent Psychiatry, 54*(2), 138–146. https://doi.org/10.1016/j.jaac.2014.10.008.

Monga, S., Young, A., & Owens, M. (2009). Evaluating a cognitive behavioral therapy group program for anxious five to seven year old children: A pilot study. *Depression and Anxiety, 26*(3), 243–250. https://doi.org/10.1002/da.20551.

Oerbeck, B., Stein, M. B., Pripp, A. H., & Kristensen, H. (2015). Selective mutism: Follow-up study 1 year after end of treatment. *European Child and Adolescent Psychiatry, 24*(7), 757–766. https://doi.org/10.1007/s00787-014-0620-1.

Pina, A. A., Silverman, W. K., Saavedra, L. M., & Weems, C. F. (2001). An analysis of the RCMAS Lie scale in a clinic sample of anxious children. *Journal of Anxiety Disorders, 15*(5), 443–457.

Pincus, D. B., Santucci, L. C., Ehrenreich, J. T., & Eyberg, S. M. (2008). The implementation of modified parent-child interaction therapy for youth with separation anxiety disorder. *Cognitive and Behavioral Practice, 15*(2), 118–125.

Reynolds, C. R., & Richmond, B. O. (1978). What I think and feel: A revised measure of children's manifest anxiety. *Journal of Abnormal Psychology, 6*(2), 271–280.

Schneider, S., Adornetto, C., & Blatter, J. (2004). *Revised children's manifest anxiety scale—Parent version (RCMAS)*. Unpublished manuscript. Switzerland: University of Basel.

Schniering, C. A., Hudson, J. L., & Rapee, R. M. (2000). Issues in the diagnosis and assessment of anxiety disorders in children and adolescents. *Clinical Psychology Review, 20*(4), 453–478.

Sharkey, L., McNicholas, F., Barry, E., Begley, M., & Ahern, S. (2008). Group therapy for selective mutism—A parents' and children's treatment group. *Journal of Behavior Therapy and Experimental Psychiatry, 39*(4), 538–545. https://doi.org/10.1016/j.jbtep.2007.12.002.

Silverman, W. K., & Albano, A. M. (1996). *The Anxiety disorders interview schedule for children for DSM-IV: Clinician manual (Child and parent versions).*

Silverman, W. K., Saavedra, L. M., & Pina, A. A. (2001). Test-retest reliability of anxiety symptoms and diagnoses with the anxiety disorders interview schedule for DSM-IV: Child and parent versions. *Journal of the American Academy of Child and Adolescent Psychiatry, 40*(8), 937–944. https://doi.org/10.1097/00004583-200108000-00016.

Spence, S. H. (1997). Structure of anxiety symptoms among children: A confirmatory factor-analytic study. *Journal of Abnormal Psychology, 106*(2), 280–297.

Spence, S. H. (1998). A measure of anxiety symptoms among children. *Behaviour Research and Therapy, 36*(5), 545–566.

Spence, S. H., & Rapee, R. (1999). *The preschool anxiety scale*. Retrieved from http://www.scaswebsite.com/docs/scas-preschool-scale.pdf.

Spence, S. H., Rapee, R., McDonald, C., & Ingram, M. (2001). The structure of anxiety symptoms among preschoolers. *Behaviour Research and Therapy, 39*, 1293–1316.

Waters, A. M., Ford, L. A., Wharton, T. A., & Cobham, V. E. (2009). Cognitive-behavioural therapy for young children with anxiety disorders: Comparison of a Child + Parent condition versus a Parent Only condition. *Behavior Research and Therapy, 47*(8), 654–662.

Chapter 3
Innovative Assessment Approaches for Young Anxious Children

3.1 Anxiety-Specific Screening Tools for Four- to Seven-Year-Old Children

3.1.1 Preschool Screen for Child Anxiety Related Emotional Disorders

The Preschool Screen for Child Anxiety Related Emotional Disorders (Pre-SCARED) is a new parent report and screening tool developed by our group to screen and identify anxiety symptoms in four- to seven-year-old children (Appendix 3.1). It is derived, with permission, from the parent version of the Screen for Child Anxiety Related Emotional Disorders (SCARED; Birmaher, Khetarpal, Brent, Cully, Balach, Kaufman, & Neer, 1997), which is a 41-item questionnaire for parents of children nine years and older (a child version that could be completed by children nine years and older is also available). The parent and child versions of the SCARED have sound psychometric properties, as established by several studies (e.g., Birmaher et al., 1997; Birmaher, Brent, Chiappetta, Bridge, Monga, & Baugher, 1999; Monga, Birmaher, Chiappetta, Brent, Kaufman, Bridge, & Cully, 2000).

The new, Pre-SCARED parent questionnaire consists of 50 items. Some items on the Pre-SCARED were taken from the SCARED and reworded in order to capture what behavior parents might observe in their young children rather than what parents might infer. For example, an item taken from the SCARED, 'When my child feels frightened it is hard for him/her to breathe' was reworded (as many parents reported not knowing if their children were having difficulty breathing or not) to become, 'When my child is frightened or scared, I notice that it is hard for him/her to breathe and/or he/she breathes rapidly.' Additionally, some items were taken from the SCARED and reworded to be more developmentally appropriate for four- to seven-year-old children. For example, the SCARED item, 'My child gets stomachaches when he/she is at school' became the Pre-SCARED item, 'My child gets stom-

© Springer Nature Switzerland AG 2018
S. Monga and D. Benoit, *Assessing and Treating Anxiety Disorders in Young Children*, https://doi.org/10.1007/978-3-030-04939-3_3

achaches when he/she is at school, daycare, or other organized activities' (as some parents of preschoolers did not answer the original SCARED question because their preschool aged children were not in school yet). Other items on the Pre-SCARED are new items, not included in, or reworded from the original SCARED. An example of a new item on the Pre-SCARED is, 'My child speaks to teachers or other caregivers when needed.' Sixteen (32%) of the current 50 items making up the Pre-SCARED were taken directly from the SCARED without modification (and with permission of the SCARED developers), 18 (36%) items were taken from the SCARED and reworded (also with permission from the SCARED creators and as described above) to be more reflective of presenting symptoms in younger children, and 16 (32%) items not found on the SCARED were newly generated.

A stepwise approach using input from clinicians experienced in preschool anxiety disorders and input from 77 parents of five- to seven-year-old children diagnosed with an anxiety disorder who completed the original parent SCARED at several time points as part of their participation in a comparative study of the Taming Sneaky Fears program (Monga, Rosenbloom, Tanha, Owens, & Young, 2015), determined which items would make up the Pre-SCARED. In the first step, items repeatedly left blank (without response), or which caused confusion (e.g., parents would ask the research coordinator how they should respond) on the original parent SCARED, were identified and discarded. In the second step, 25 (33%) of the 77 parents provided specific and detailed feedback as to which items from the SCARED they felt were relevant (or applied to their anxious five- to seven-year-old children), and which were not. In the third step, experienced clinicians provided their impressions as to whether the items from the original SCARED that were retained in the Pre-SCARED were relevant anxiety symptoms for young children and were appropriately worded (or reworded) for parents of younger children. In the fourth step, as our goal was to generate about 50 items for the Pre-SCARED, clinicians experienced in preschool anxiety disorders generated new items for inclusion in the Pre-SCARED, targeting anxiety symptoms that were not already included on the Pre-SCARED; consensus among the experienced clinicians yielded several new items pertaining to social anxiety and selective mutism. In the fifth and final step, parent feedback about the original SCARED not providing enough choices of responses (with the SCARED three-point rating scale), guided the decision to use a five-point scale (0 = never, 1 = almost never, 2 = sometimes, 3 = almost always, and 4 = always). Appendix 3.1 provides the 50 items from the Pre-SCARED. As with the SCARED, the Pre-SCARED yields one total score, which is derived from a total summation of the rating scores on each of the 50 items.

Efforts to validate the new Pre-SCARED to aid in the screening of young children presenting with symptoms or concerns of anxiety are ongoing. Early evidence suggests that this 50-item screen is internally consistent, with Cronbach's $\alpha = 0.94$, based on Pre-SCARED data obtained from 224 parents of four- to seven-year-old children (M age = 5.6 years; $SD = 1.1$; 102 males) presenting to our clinic for a new psychiatric assessment (67% were given an anxiety disorder diagnosis, 19% were given a non-anxiety disorder diagnosis, 13% were not given any psychiatric diagnosis). A subsample ($N = 113$) completed both the Pre-SCARED and the Preschool

Anxiety Scale (Spence & Rapee, 1999), which, as discussed in Chap. 2, is a widely used screening tool used with parents of young children. The correlation between the Pre-SCARED total score and the Preschool Anxiety Scale total score was $r = 0.81$, $p < 0.001$, suggesting convergent validity of the Pre-SCARED with the Preschool Anxiety Scale.

Further evaluation of the psychometric properties of the Pre-SCARED is currently under way.

3.2 Tools to Assess Selective Mutism and Social Anxiety Disorder

As described in Chap. 2, there are currently few well-validated, user-friendly instruments to reliably assess symptoms of anxiety in four- to seven-year-old children, and even fewer well-validated, user-friendly tools available to reliably assess selective mutism and/or social anxiety disorder in this age group. As part of a recently completed data collection phase of a randomized control trial comparing the efficacy of two group interventions in the treatment of four- to seven-year-old children with selective mutism and/or social anxiety disorder and their parents ($N = 94$; M age $= 5.44$ years; $SD = 1.0$; 28 males) (Sect. 5.3.5), our research group developed four novel instruments to assist clinicians and researchers in the assessment of these conditions. These novel assessment tools include the Mutism Accommodation Scale, the Talking Behavior Assessment Tool, the Selective Mutism Versus Social Anxiety Disorder Criteria Checklist and the Steps to Talking. Preliminary data regarding these novel tools show promise in both the clinical and research assessments of four- to seven-year-old children presenting with the symptom of 'not speaking' or possible selective mutism and/or social anxiety disorder. These assessment tools and their suggested use in the assessment process are discussed below. As most of these assessment tools were recently developed, extensive psychometric evaluation is pending. Whenever relevant and feasible, preliminary results regarding psychometric properties of these instruments are provided.

3.2.1 Mutism Accommodation Scale

The Mutism Accommodation Scale (Appendix 3.2) is a 22-item parent questionnaire that was developed on the premise that parents and caregivers could unintentionally accommodate their children's mutism in order to alleviate their children's distress. For example, parents of children with selective mutism may speak or allow others to speak for their children, allow or facilitate non-verbal communication instead of verbal communication, and even allow their children to avoid distressing situations in which speech is expected. In children with non-specific anxiety disorders, such forms of accommodation have been associated with increased symptom severity, lower levels of functioning, and poorer outcomes (Thompson-Hollands, Kerns, Pincus, & Comer, 2014). Although not studied previously in selective mutism, parental accommodation may have a contributory role in the development and maintenance of selective mutism. As such, the items for the Mutism Accommodation Scale were generated based upon other scales of accommodation that have been used in various psychiatric disorders such as obsessive-compulsive disorder. Our hypothesis is that parental accommodation would decrease as the children's selective mutism improves with treatment. This is a hypothesis that has partial support based on preliminary evidence with parents who completed the Taming Sneaky Fears Cognitive Behavior Therapy program (Chaps. 5–11), which encourages parents to set a clear expectation for speech and supportively push their children past their fear of being seen and heard speaking by Climbing Bravery Ladders for speaking (gradual exposure or progressive desensitization; see Chap. 10 for further details). However, an equally valid hypothesis is that a decrease in parental accommodation would result in an improvement in child's speaking behavior. As part of our randomized control trial (data collection recently completed), all parents completed the Mutism Accommodation Scale at all assessment time points (Sect. 5.3.5). Data analyses are underway and we plan to examine the question of what comes first, a reduction in parental accommodation or an improvement in the child's speaking behavior.

3.2.2 Talking Behavior Assessment Tool

The Talking Behavior Assessment Tool (Appendix 3.3) is a clinician-administered tool that was developed as an interview guide for clinicians and researchers when conducting assessment interviews with parents of four- to seven-year-old children who present with the symptom of 'not speaking' or who are referred for possible selective mutism and/or social anxiety disorder.

As seen in Appendix 3.3, the Talking Behavior Assessment Tool inquires about the number and variety of languages spoken at home, the child's comfort level with different languages (if applicable), as well as whether parents note concerns with their child's speech and language skills. Additionally, the Talking Behavior Assessment Tool inquires about the child's speaking behavior and level of verbal interaction in a variety of settings (e.g., home, daycare, school, and community). As clinicians or researchers interview the parents, a checkmark indicating the child's best performance in each specific setting or situation or with each specific individual is noted. Such a tool provides a detailed, structured, and consistent approach when asking about a child's speaking behaviors in a variety of settings. The Talking Behavior Assessment Tool is currently used in our clinic on a regular basis. It is used primarily for descriptive and qualitative purposes.

3.2.3 Selective Mutism Versus Social Anxiety Disorder Criteria Checklist

As discussed in Chap. 1, the extant literature on anxiety disorders documents the high comorbidity of selective mutism and social anxiety disorder. As reviewed in Chap. 2, there are few standardized tools that currently exist to assess the specific symptoms characterizing selective mutism. Because of this high comorbidity and the lack of validated measures to assess selective mutism, it is often difficult to distinguish between the symptoms that characterize selective mutism and social anxiety disorder and thus difficult to untangle which is the primary diagnosis when a young child presents with the symptom of 'not speaking.' Our research group developed the Selective Mutism Versus Social Anxiety Criteria Checklist (Appendix 3.4) for clinicians and researchers to use during a clinical assessment to evaluate whether the child's symptom of 'not speaking' reflects a primary diagnosis of selective mutism, social anxiety disorder, or both.

The Selective Mutism Versus Social Anxiety Criteria Checklist consists of two subscales, a selective mutism subscale and a social anxiety disorder subscale, each of which includes three items that capture the core features or characteristics of each disorder. After completing a clinical assessment and interview with the child who is a potential research subject and/or presents in clinic with the symptom of 'not speaking,' the clinician or researcher uses a four-point scale (0 = don't know/not sure; 1 = false or no; 2 = variable; and 3 = true or yes) to rate each of the six items on the checklist. The score for each subscale ranges from 0 to 9. The first item for each subscale (item 1 and item 4) focuses on the 'warm up' time required for a child to speak in school or other social settings. Clinicians and researchers keep in mind that when evaluating young children who are not speaking at school with teachers, it is necessary to consider the child's age and the time of the school year when the assessment is taking place. For example, if a child presenting for an assessment in March has not been speaking to the teacher since the beginning of the school year in September, a diagnosis of selective mutism is likely (assuming that other psychiatric diagnoses have been ruled out as explanations for not speaking). Conversely, a child presenting for an assessment in October (shortly after the start of the school year) could have either social anxiety disorder or selective mutism as it is yet unclear whether the child might 'warm up' and begin to speak if given enough 'warm up' time.

Items 2 and 3 of the Selective Mutism Versus Social Anxiety Criteria Checklist (selective mutism subscale) focus on the observations that many children with a primary diagnosis of selective mutism are able to interact in a more normative fashion if they are not required to speak. Items 5 and 6 on the Selective Mutism Versus Social Anxiety Criteria Checklist (social anxiety disorder subscale) focus on the observations that children with a primary diagnosis of social anxiety disorder typically demonstrate self-consciousness (e.g., worries about embarrassment or being judged) and physical signs of tension, which typically would not be seen in children with 'pure' selective mutism.

Clinical experience with the Selective Mutism Versus Social Anxiety Criteria Checklist suggests that if a clinician rates most of items 1–3 as 'true/yes or variable' and most of items 4–6 as 'false/no,' the child is likely to have a primary diagnosis of selective mutism. Conversely, if a clinician rates most of items 4–6 as 'true/yes or variable' and most of items 1–3 as 'false/no,' the child is likely to have a primary diagnosis of social anxiety disorder. Children receiving high scores on all six items of the Selective Mutism Versus Social Anxiety Criteria Checklist likely have co-morbid selective mutism and social anxiety disorder requiring the clinician to evaluate which is the primary diagnosis based upon the use of other tools and clinical judgment.

Both the Selective Mutism Versus Social Anxiety Criteria Checklist and the Anxiety Disorders Interview Schedule Parent version (Silverman & Albano, 1996), a well-validated semi-structured interview used for diagnostic purposes in many preschool anxiety research trials (as discussed in Chap. 2), were completed in a sample of four- to seven-year-old children ($N = 84$; M age $= 5.83$ years; $SD = 1.11$; 25 males) attending our clinic for an assessment of selective mutism and/or social anxiety disorder. Using Spearman correlations, the selective mutism subscale of the Selective Mutism Versus Social Anxiety Criteria Checklist correlated significantly with the Anxiety Disorders Interview Schedule Parent version—Clinician Severity Rating for selective mutism ($r_s = 0.52$, $p < 0.001$), while the social anxiety disorder subscale of the Selective Mutism Versus Social Anxiety Criteria Checklist correlated significantly with the Anxiety Disorders Interview Schedule Parent version—Clinician Severity Rating for social anxiety disorder ($r_s = 0.43$, $p < 0.001$). These findings provide preliminary convergent validity of the Selective Mutism Versus Social Anxiety Criteria Checklist.

Clinical experience and preliminary data provide some support that the Selective Mutism Versus Social Anxiety Criteria Checklist could assist clinicians and researchers in distinguishing between a diagnosis of selective mutism and social anxiety disorder, or establishing co-morbidity of the two diagnoses in young children who present with a symptom of not speaking. Further validation and exploration of the psychometric properties of this tool are warranted and are currently underway.

3.2.4 Steps to Talking

The Steps to Talking (Appendix 3.5) is a novel clinician-administered instrument that can be used by clinicians and researchers in the assessment of four- to seven-year-old children presenting for 'not speaking' or possible selective mutism and/or social anxiety disorder. The Steps to Talking quantify a child's nonverbal and verbal communication with an assessor during an encounter. The level of nonverbal and verbal interaction is measured at three time points during a clinical encounter: (1) immediately upon greeting; (2) within the first 30 minutes of the encounter; and

(3) any time after the first 30 minutes of the encounter. As seen in Appendix 3.5, the clinician or researcher indicates in the first column the child's highest or best (between 1 and 16) verbal or nonverbal performance immediately when first greeting the child. The clinician or researcher then indicates in the second column the child's highest or best (between 1 and 16) verbal or nonverbal performance with the assessor within the first 30 minutes of an encounter. The clinician or researcher then uses the third column to indicate the child's highest or best (between 1 and 16) verbal or nonverbal performance with the assessor any time after the first 30 minutes of the encounter.

For example, a child who comes in for an assessment might only nod to the assessor in the waiting room when first greeted and not move beyond nodding within the first 30 minutes and beyond. As seen in Appendix 3.5, that child would receive a score of 5 in the 'Immediately upon greeting' column, a score of 5 in the 'Within the first 30 minutes.' column, and a score of 5 in the 'Any time after 30 minutes.' column, and thus would not demonstrate any change over the course of the encounter in the level of verbal (or nonverbal) interaction. This child would likely have selective mutism as clinical experience with the Steps to Talking tool suggests that the ratings for children with selective mutism appear to remain flat across the three time points during an encounter with an assessor.

Conversely, a child might hide behind a parent's leg and only make fleeting eye contact when first greeted in the waiting room and might be able to nod and use various gestures in response to questions during the first 30 minutes. With further warm up time beyond the first 30 minutes, that same child, who was not speaking at the start of the interview, may respond to questions from the assessor using two- to four-word responses with a normal volume voice. On the Steps to Talking this child's scores would be 3 in the 'Immediately upon greeting' column, 5 in the 'Within the first 30 minutes.' column, and 14 in the 'Any time after 30 minutes.' column. This child likely has social anxiety disorder as clinical experience with the Steps to Talking suggests that children with social anxiety disorder show an upward progression of scores over the course of the encounter as the child warms up.

To formally test the hypotheses (derived from the aforementioned clinical experience) that a flat line (or near flat line) across the three time points on the Steps to Talking is characteristic of young children with selective mutism, while an upward progression of scores across the three time points is characteristic of young children with social anxiety disorder, we conducted a cluster analysis on the data collected in the sample of 94 four- to seven-year-old children (M age $= 5.44$ years; $SD = 1.0$; 28 males) with selective mutism and/or anxiety disorder who consented to participate in the recently completed randomized control trial and for which data were available (Sect. 5.3.5). To identify a priori profiles and following implementation of the k-means algorithm (Genolini, Alacoque, Sentenac, & Arnaud, 2015) and the Calinski and Harabasz criterion (1974), three clusters were identified (Fig. 3.1): Cluster A included patients with consistently low scores ($N = 41$), Cluster B included those with overall increasing scores ($N = 36$), and Cluster C included those with consistently high scores ($N = 17$).

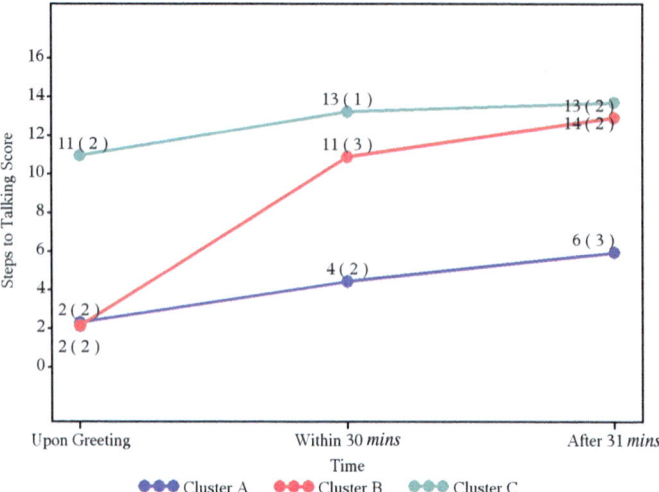

Fig. 3.1 Cluster analysis of mean Steps to Talking scores (standard deviation) over three time points; *Mins* minutes

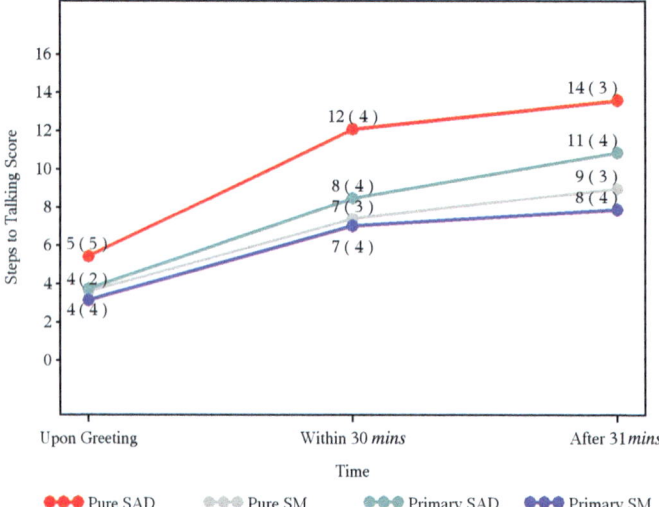

Fig. 3.2 Cluster analysis of mean Steps to Talking scores (standard deviation) over three time points by diagnostic group; *SAD* social anxiety disorder; *SM* selective mutism; *Mins* minutes

Additionally, a cluster analysis using data from the same sample was performed based upon four diagnostic groups: (1) 'pure' selective mutism; (2) primary selective mutism plus social anxiety disorder; (3) primary social anxiety disorder plus selective mutism; and (4) 'pure' social anxiety disorder (Fig. 3.2).

And finally, using a logistic regression analyses, clusters A, B, and C (Fig. 3.1) were found to be associated with diagnosis, with the odds of 'pure' selective mutism or primary selective mutism diagnoses being 5.6 (95% CI: 2.3–14.1, $p < 0.001$) times higher in cluster A compared to clusters B + C.

As implied from the aforementioned examples, and based on clinical observation and preliminary research evidence, the Steps to Talking tool shows promise as a user-friendly tool that could, in a single one-hour encounter, assist clinicians and researchers in distinguishing selective mutism from social anxiety disorder in young children, and could potentially be used to monitor children's progress in using their voice to speak during treatment or intervention studies.

3.3 Future Directions and Goals

Given the paucity of validated screening and assessment tools developed specifically for use with four- to seven-year old children with anxiety disorders as discussed in Chap. 2, our clinical research group has been actively engaged in the development and validation of new and innovative tools to screen and assess anxiety disorders in young children, with a special focus on selective mutism and social anxiety disorder. To date, our group has developed five tools specifically for use with four- to seven-year-old children with anxiety disorders in clinical and research settings. These tools require additional refinement and more thorough psychometric evaluation and validation, which is currently under way. We presented herein a snapshot of the early theoretical framework and psychometric data, where relevant and available, for these novel tools. We welcome having clinicians and researchers use and further refine these tools.

Appendix 3.1

Child's Name/ID _____   Date: _____

PRE-SCHOOL SCREEN FOR CHILDHOOD ANXIETY RELATED DISORDERS (Pre-SCARED)
Parent Form
Monga, S. & Benoit, D. (2017)

Below is a list of items that describe how children may feel. Read each statement carefully and place a check mark (✓) in the box that best reflects how often your child displays each of the behavior described below. Please answer all items as well as you can, even if some do not seem to concern your child.

		Never	Almost never	Sometimes	Almost always	Always
1	When my child is frightened or scared, I notice that it is hard for him/her to breathe and/or he/she breathes rapidly					
2	My child gets headaches when he/she is at school, daycare, or other organized activities					
3	My child quickly feels comfortable with people he/she doesn't know well					
4	My child speaks to teachers or other caregivers when needed					
5	My child worries about other people liking him/her					
6	When my child gets frightened or scared, I notice that he/she looks flushed					
7	My child is nervous					
8	My child follows me wherever I go (he/she is like my shadow)					
9	People tell me that my child looks nervous					
10	My child feels nervous with people he/she doesn't know well					
11	My child gets stomach aches at school, daycare, or other organized activities					
12	My child worries about things that might happen in the future					
13	My child is able to fall asleep on his/her own					
14	My child worries about being as good as other kids					
15	When my child gets frightened or scared, I notice that he/she acts out or has an angry meltdown					
16	My child has nightmares about something bad happening to his/her parents (e.g., getting lost/ kidnapped, injury, accident, death)					
17	My child worries about going to school, daycare, or other organized activities					

		Never	Almost never	Sometimes	Almost always	Always
18	When my child gets frightened or scared, I notice that his/her heart beats fast					
19	When my child gets frightened or scared, I notice that he/she shakes or trembles					
20	My child has nightmares about something bad happening to him/her (e.g., getting lost/kidnapped, injury, accident, death)					
21	My child worries more about things than most children his/her age					
22	When my child gets frightened or scared, I notice that he/she sweats a lot					
23	My child is a worrier					
24	My child gets really frightened or scared for no reason at all					
25	My child is afraid to be alone in an area of the house (e.g., basement, bedroom)					
26	It is hard for my child to talk with people he/she doesn't know well					
27	When my child gets frightened or scared, he/she feels like he/she is choking					
28	People tell me that my child worries too much					
29	My child doesn't like to be away from his/her family					
30	My child worries that their own voice will be too loud					
31	My child gets upset when I leave him/her with another caregiver (e.g., babysitter, grandparent, teacher)					
32	My child worries that something bad might happen to his/her parents					
33	My child feels shy with adults he/she doesn't know well					
34	My child feels shy with children he/she doesn't know well					
35	My child needs to be given a lot of explanations and/or reassurance about things that are going to happen					
36	When my child gets frightened or scared, he/she feels like throwing up					
37	My child worries that their own voice will sound funny					
38	My child worries about how well he/she does things					

		Never	Almost never	Sometimes	Almost always	Always
39	When my child meets new people, he/she becomes quieter than usual for a while after first meeting the new people, but then warms up					
40	My child worries about things that have already happened					
41	When my child meets new people, he/she becomes quieter than usual for the whole time he/she is with the new people					
42	My child feels nervous when he/she is with other children or adults and has to do something while they watch him/her (for example: read aloud, speak, play a game, or play a sport)					
43	My child feels nervous about going to birthday parties or any place where there will be people that he/she doesn't know well					
44	My child worries that adults and/ or children will laugh at him/her					
45	My child is shy					
46	My child speaks to many peers without difficulty					
47	My child dislikes having attention drawn to him/her					
48	My child worries about trying a new activity					
49	My child is scared to go to school, daycare, or other organized activities					
50	My child has trouble controlling his/her worries					

Appendix 3.2

Child's Name/ID _____   Date: _____

Mutism Accommodation Scale (MARS: Parent Version)
Monga, S. & Benoit, D. (2017)

Below is a list of items that describe what parents do when their child does not speak or speaks very little in various social situations. Read each statement carefully and place a check mark (✓) in the box that best reflects how often you do each item. If an item does not apply to you, please place a check mark (✓) in the N/A (Not Applicable) box. Please answer all items as well as you can, even if some do not seem to concern you.

		Never	Almost never	Sometimes	Almost always	Always	N/A
1	I avoid social situations because my child will become upset or "shut down."						
2	I arrange play dates and other social interactions for my child						

In various social situations (e.g., school, play dates, birthday parties, extra-curricular activities, camps, visits with extended family):		Never	Almost never	Sometimes	Almost always	Always	N/A
3	I speak for my child						
4	I allow my child's siblings to speak for him/her						
5	I become anxious when my child does not speak, so I don't expect or encourage him/her to speak						
6	I tell people my child is shy						
7	I allow my child to whisper to others						
8	I tell my child that he/she does not have to speak						
9	I encourage other children (e.g., classmates, peers) to speak for my child						
10	I praise or reward my child when he/she speaks						
11	I become angry, annoyed, or frustrated when my child does not speak so, I don't expect or encourage him/her to speak						
12	I tell teachers, coaches, and other adults that my child does not speak						
13	I am surprised (shocked) when my child speaks to adults he/she does not know well						
14	I am surprised (shocked) when my child speaks to children he/she does not know well						
15	I know my child will become upset or "shut down" when he/she has to speak, so I don't expect or encourage my child to speak						
16	I allow my child to nod, use other gestures, or facial expressions instead of his/her voice						
17	I encourage other adults (e.g., nanny, babysitter, grandparents) to speak for my child						
18	I allow my child to whisper answers to me						
19	I become embarrassed when my child does not speak, so I don't expect or encourage my child to speak						

In various social situations (e.g., school, play dates, birthday parties, extra-curricular activities, camps, visits with extended family):	Never	Almost never	Sometimes	Almost always	Always	N/A
20	I apologize to adults or children for my child not talking						
21	I allow my child to say parts of words or sounds instead of saying a full word						
22	I whisper to my child						

Appendix 3.3

Child's Name/ID _____   Coder: _____   Date: _____

TALKING BEHAVIOR ASSESSMENT TOOL
Benoit, D. & Monga S. (2017)

Languages spoken at home: English___   Other: _____

Main language spoken at home: English___   Other: _____

Language child most comfortable speaking: English___   Other: _____

Concern about speech, articulation, etc.: _____

Place a checkmark to indicate the child's best performance with respect to ability to communicate in the following settings:

Home:

	Nothing (no gesture and no voice)	Gestures	Whisper	Soft voice	Normal volume voice	How long a warm up period is needed before speaking
Parents						
Siblings						
Extended family						
Family friends						
Babysitter						
Visitors (strangers)						
Other						

Day care:

	Nothing (no gesture and no voice)	Gestures	Whisper	Soft voice	Normal volume voice	How long a warm up period is needed before speaking
Close friends						
Children						
Primary caregiver						
Other caregiver						
Other						

School:

	Nothing (no gesture and no voice)	Gestures	Whisper	Soft voice	Normal volume voice	How long a warm up period is needed before speaking
Close friends						
Children						
Classroom teacher						
Other adult						
Concert/play/ show & tell						
Other						
Other						

Community:

	Nothing (no gesture and no voice)	Gestures	Whisper	Soft voice	Normal volume voice	How long a warm up period is needed before speaking
Neighbors – children						
Neighbors – adults						
Play date – close friend						
Play date – parent(s) of close friend						
Extra-curricular activity – close friend						
Extra-curricular activity – other children						
Extra-curricular activity – coach						
Restaurant – waiter / waitress						
Stores – cashier / store employee						
Park – children						
Park – adult						
Doctor / dentist / optometrist						
Other						
Other						

Appendix 3.4

Child's Name/ID _____   Coder: _____   Date: _____

Selective Mutism vs. Social Anxiety Disorder Criteria Checklist
Monga, S. & Benoit, D. (2017)

		Score	3	2	1	0
			True or Yes	Variable (sometimes true, sometimes false)	False or No	Don't know, not specified, or not applicable
Selective Mutism if most/all of criteria #1 – 3 are True or Variable	1	Will not speak to a specific person or specific people, or in one (or more) specific setting(s), even after a warm-up period				
	2	During activities (e.g., extra-curricular activities, gym class, performances), participates non-verbally without difficulty, but remains non-verbal when speech is expected				
	3	With peers, interacts socially, but non-verbally				
		Count the totals of each column	**Total Selective Mutism Score**			
	4	Will interact, participate, (or speak), but only after a warm-up period				
[a] **Social Anxiety Disorder** if most/all of criteria #4 – 6 are True or Variable	5	Conveys self-consciousness (e.g., worries about being embarrassed, made fun of, laughed at, in the spotlight, or having attention focused on him/her, whether perceived or actual)				
	6	Displays physical signs of tension (e.g., shoulders hunched, wringing hands, downward gaze, hiding behind parent) in most social encounters, whether in groups or one-on-one, including with assessor				
		Count the totals of each column	**Total Social Anxiety Disorder Score**			

[a] Anxiety about being observed or scrutinized must be present with adults and peers.

Appendix 3.5

Child's ID _____ Coder: _____ Date: _____

STEPS TO TALKING
for Selective Mutism and Social Anxiety Disorder
Monga, S. & Benoit, D. (2017)

How long was today's assessment? _____ hours
(i.e., how long was the observation that yielded the ratings below)

This checklist is to be completed by an assessor after spending at least one hour completing an assessment with the child, in the presence of the child's primary caregiver(s). Circle the number corresponding to the highest step achieved by the child during interactions with the assessor (unless otherwise specified) within each time point during the period of observation.

Steps to talking		Immediately upon greeting	Within the first 30 minutes of encounter	Any time after 30 minutes	
11	Spontaneously asks questions or volunteers information (soft or normal voice) to assessor	16	16	16	
10	Responds to questions ($\geq$ 5 words normal voice) to assessor	15	15	15	
9	2-4 word response(s) with normal voice to assessor	14	14	14	
8	1 word response(s) with normal voice (e.g. only yes, no) to assessor	13	13	13	
7	> 1 word spoken in soft voice with assessor	12	12	12	
6	> 1 word response(s) in (soft / normal – circle one) voice with (parent / other:_____ - circle one)	11	11	11	
5	1 word responses in soft voice only (e.g., yes, no) to assessor	10	10	10	
4	1 word responses in soft voice only (e.g., yes, no) to parent / other	9	9	9	
3	$\geq$ 1 word(s) whispered *audibly* to assessor	8	8	8	
2	$\geq$ 1 word(s) whispered *audibly* to parent/ other	7	7	7	
1	Mouths $\geq$ 1 word(s)	6	6	6	
	Nods or gestures, spontaneously or upon request, to respond to the assessor's questions	5	5	5	
	Sustains eye contact with the assessor	4	4	4	
	Makes fleeting eye contact with the assessor	3	3	3	
	Positions self to be face to face with assessor	2	2	2	
	Willing to be in the same room with assessor	1	1	1	0

Notes: _____

References

Birmaher, B., Brent, D. A., Chiappetta, L., Bridge, J., Monga, S., & Baugher, M. (1999). Psychometric properties of the Screen for Child Anxiety Related Emotional Disorders (SCARED): A replication study. *Journal of the American Academy of Child and Adolescent Psychiatry, 38*(10), 1230–1236. https://doi.org/10.1097/00004583-199910000-00011.

Birmaher, B., Khetarpal, S., Brent, D., Cully, M., Balach, L., Kaufman, J., & Neer, S. M. (1997). The Screen for Child Anxiety Related Emotional Disorders (SCARED): Scale construction and psychometric characteristics. *Journal of the American Academy of Child and Adolescent Psychiatry, 36*(4), 545–553. https://doi.org/10.1097/00004583-199704000-00018.

Calinski, T., & Harabasz, J. (1974). A dendrite method for cluster analysis. *Communications in Statistics, 3*(1), 1–27.

Genolini, C., Alacoque, X., Sentenac, M., & Arnaud, C. (2015). Kml and kml3d: R packages to cluster longitudinal data. *Journal of Statistical Software, 65*(4), 1–34. URL http://www.jstatsoft.org/v65/i04/.

Monga, S., Birmaher, B., Chiappetta, L., Brent, D., Kaufman, J., Bridge, J., & Cully, M. (2000). Screen for Child Anxiety-Related Emotional Disorders (SCARED): Convergent and divergent validity. *Depression and Anxiety, 12*(2), 85–91. https://doi.org/10.1002/1520-6394(2000)12:2%3c85::aid-da4%3e3.0.co;2-2.

Monga, S., Rosenbloom, B. N., Tanha, A., Owens, M., & Young, A. (2015). Comparison of child-parent and parent-only cognitive-behavioral therapy programs for anxious children aged 5 to 7 years: Short- and long-term outcomes. *Journal of the American Academy of Child and Adolescent Psychiatry, 54*(2), 138–146. https://doi.org/10.1016/j.jaac.2014.10.008.

Silverman, W. K. & Albano, A. M. (1996). *The Anxiety disorders interview schedule for children for DSM-IV: Clinician manual (Child and parent versions).*

Spence, S. H., & Rapee, R. (1999). *The preschool anxiety scale.* Retrieved from http://www.scaswebsite.com/docs/scas-preschool-scale.pdf.

Thompson-Hollands, J., Kerns, C. E., Pincus, D. B., & Comer, J. S. (2014). Parental accommodation of child anxiety and related symptoms: Range, impact, and correlates. *Journal of Anxiety Disorders, 28*(8), 765–773. https://doi.org/10.1016/j.janxdis.2014.09.007.

Chapter 4
Current Evidence-Based Management

4.1 Introduction

As evident from Chaps. 1 and 2, the current state of knowledge about preschool anxiety disorders is in its infancy, and this is also reflected in the paucity of research studies on the treatment of anxiety disorders in young children. Early beliefs were that young anxious children were too developmentally immature and cognitively unsophisticated to take an active part in any treatment program and therefore, early treatment approaches were primarily parent-focused. However, in the last decade, two main therapeutic approaches, Parent-Child Interaction Therapy and Cognitive Behavior Therapy (CBT) have directly involved young anxious children in treatment sessions. The fundamental philosophies of these two approaches, however, are quite different, with the focus of Parent-Child Interaction Therapy being on the parent-child relationship while the focus of CBT is on the individual child's recognition of the links among thought, feeling, and behavior. Therefore, these two types of interventions are described as distinct in this chapter even though Parent-Child Interaction Therapy for preschool anxiety disorders has incorporated behavioral strategies borrowed from CBT (Sect. 4.2) and as a result a similar behavioral focus and use of exposure hierarchies characterize both CBT approaches with preschool children and Parent-Child Interaction Therapy, thus making these two types of interventions more similar than dissimilar in the management of preschool anxiety disorders (Sect. 4.3). Finally, the various approaches, again primarily behavioral, that have been used with selective mutism, are discussed in Sect. 4.4.

© Springer Nature Switzerland AG 2018
S. Monga and D. Benoit, *Assessing and Treating Anxiety Disorders in Young Children*, https://doi.org/10.1007/978-3-030-04939-3_4

4.2 Parent-Child Interaction Therapy

Parent-Child Interaction Therapy is a dyadic behavioral intervention developed by Eyberg and her colleagues for two- to seven-year-old children and their caregivers (Brinkmeyer & Eyberg, 2003). Its primary focus is to decrease externalizing child behavior problems, increase child social skills and cooperation, and improve parent-child relationship and interaction patterns. To date, Parent-Child Interaction Therapy has been used primarily in the management of disruptive behavioral disorders with an established evidence base in this population (e.g., Eyberg et al., 2001; Eyberg, Nelson, & Boggs, 2008; Hood & Eyberg, 2003). A typical course of Parent-Child Interaction Therapy consists of about 14 weekly, one-hour sessions. Parent-Child Interaction Therapy has two main components, Child-Directed Interaction and Parent-Directed Interaction. In the initial Child-Directed Interaction component, the focus is on developing a warm and nurturing bond between parents and children through play. This is followed by the Parent-Directed Interaction component in which, through the use of play therapy and behavioral therapy, parents learn more effective ways of disciplining their children. Given the evidence for its efficacy in helping two- to seven-year-old children with behavioral difficulties, Parent-Child Interaction Therapy was adapted for use in the management of anxiety disorders in this same age group in more recent years.

In an open trial pilot study, Pincus, Santucci, Ehrenreich, and Eyberg (2008) utilized Parent-Child Interaction Therapy with ten children (M age = 6.2 years; range = 4–8) with separation anxiety disorder diagnosed using the Anxiety Disorders Interview Schedule (Silverman & Albano, 1996). Although mean Anxiety Disorders Interview Schedule Clinician Severity Rating decreased from 5.8 pre-treatment to 4.2 post-treatment (no p values were reported), they did not decrease below non-clinical levels (as described in Chap. 2, a Clinician Severity Rating of 4 or greater on the Anxiety Disorders Interview Schedule indicates a clinical diagnosis). Additionally, according to Pincus and colleagues (2008), although improvements in separation symptoms were noted in practiced situations, children continued to have difficulties with separation in new situations. Given these early findings, Pincus and colleagues (2008) added a third component, they called Bravery-Directed Interaction, which is further described in Sect. 4.2.1.

4.2.1 Bravery-Directed Interaction

Similar to the Child-Directed Interaction and Parent-Directed Interaction components of traditional Parent-Child Interaction Therapy, the Bravery-Directed Interaction component consists of one Teach session for parents followed by two or more Coach sessions. Psychoeducation about anxiety, factors that maintain anxiety, and links among thoughts, physical feelings, and behaviors is provided during this Teach session. Additionally, therapists help parents build fear and avoidance hierarchies and reward lists, demonstrate how to complete and practice hierarchies with their children outside of sessions, and discuss the importance of using Child-Directed Interaction skills (e.g., praising brave behaviors and reflecting on emotions and behaviors) and avoiding avoidance during the Teach session. Coach sessions follow in which therapists 'coach' parents on ways to develop exposure practices during the week between therapy sessions, as well as problem solve around exposures already conducted. The Bravery-Directed Interaction component uses CBT-like principles, although it maintains the same behavioral focus of traditional Parent-Child Interaction Therapy.

Pincus and colleagues presented preliminary data on a randomized control trial of the Bravery-Directed Interaction (Pincus et al., 2008; Puliafico, Comer, & Pincus, 2012) component of Parent-Child Interaction Therapy in which 38 four- to eight-year-old children (15 males; no additional demographic data provided) with a primary diagnosis of separation anxiety disorder were randomized to either the Bravery-Directed Interaction arm or a 9-week waitlist control arm after which time the children received the active treatment. They report that the parent-child dyads who received the modified Parent-Child Interaction Therapy had greater improvements on separation anxiety, general psychopathology, parent-child interaction, and parent stress than those in the waitlist control arm at post-treatment, with 73% of children no longer meeting diagnostic criteria for separation anxiety disorder post-treatment, and these improvements were maintained at a 12-month follow-up visit (Puliafico et al., 2012). Further data from this randomized control trial would be necessary to fully evaluate the efficacy of Parent-Child Interaction Therapy and the modified CBT-like Bravery-Directed Interaction in the treatment of preschool anxiety disorders, but no such data have been published. Although the aforementioned preliminary data suggest that Bravery-Directed Interaction, a modification of Parent-Child Interaction Therapy, may be helpful in the treatment of separation anxiety disorder, further evaluation with larger sample sizes and more rigorous methodology is needed.

4.2.2 Coaching Approach Behavior and Leading by Modeling

Another anxiety-focused modification of Parent-Child Interaction Therapy designed to treat young children with several different anxiety disorders, including separation anxiety disorder, social anxiety disorder, generalized anxiety disorder, or specific phobia, is the Coaching Approach Behavior and Leading by Modeling (CALM) program (Comer, Puliafico, Aschenbrand, McKnight, Robin, Goldfin, & Albano, 2012). In this modification of Parent-Child Interaction Therapy, the Child-Directed Interaction component remains unchanged, the Parent-Directed Interaction component is omitted, and the CALM program, a 12-session manual-based modification, is added. In the CALM program, the foci in four initial Child-Directed Interaction sessions are the parent-child relationship, psychoeducation about anxiety, and the development of fear hierarchies. This is followed by eight exposure sessions during which parents complete exposure tasks with their children while wearing an in-ear earbud that allows them to hear and receive real-time, in-session coaching or individualized feedback. The CALM program emphasizes parent modeling of approach behaviors for the child, setting clear expectations about the child's behavior, using effective communication with the child in anxiety-provoking situations, and using praise following the child's display of brave behaviors while ignoring behaviors such as avoidance and whining. The CALM program's developers emphasize that the individualized, real-time feedback via the earbud in the parent's ear during sessions distinguishes this program from other CBT-like programs that utilize exposure (Comer et al., 2012).

Nine children (*M* age = 5.4 years; *SD* = 1.3; range = 4–8) with a primary anxiety disorder diagnosis (separation anxiety disorder, social anxiety disorder, or specific phobia), established by the Anxiety Disorders Interview Schedule (Silverman & Albano, 1996), participated with their parents in a pilot study of the CALM program (Comer et al., 2012). Children with a moderate degree of interference, as measured by a score of less than 55 on the Children's Global Assessment Scale (Shaffer, Gould, Brasic, Ambrosini, Fisher, Bird, & Aluwahlia, 1983), were excluded. The Children's Global Assessment Scale is a clinician rating of overall functioning rated on a 100-point scale with higher scores reflecting higher adaptive functioning. No changes in the Anxiety Disorders Interview Schedule Clinician Severity Rating or the Children's Global Assessment Scale were noted between two baseline assessments conducted by independent assessors one to four weeks apart. Two of the nine children dropped out of treatment early. Using an intent-to-treat analysis, six (66.7%) of the nine children no longer met criteria for any diagnosis post-treatment. A mean Anxiety Disorders Interview Schedule Clinician Severity Rating decrease of 2.8 (*SD* = 2.0) for the primary diagnosis was noted (no *p* value reported). Additionally, a mean improvement in the Children's Global Assessment Scale of 21 points (*SD* = 11 points) was noted (no *p* value reported), with six (66.7%) of the nine children categorized as having a functional improvement of at least 10 points, or movement from one interval on the Children's Global Assessment Scale to the next interval, which would be clinically significant (Shaffer et al., 1983).

Comer et al. (2012) hypothesized that direct modifications in parenting practices and parenting reinforcement contingencies were responsible for the improvements noted in the six children. Although this small open trial pilot study provides preliminary support for this modified approach to Parent-Child Interaction Therapy and suggests that reshaping parenting practices may be helpful in reducing children's anxiety, significant study limitations must be highlighted. For example, the small sample size and the fact that children with significant impairment (i.e., those with Children's Global Assessment Scale scores of less than 55) were excluded from participating in the study are significant limitations. In fact, the pre-treatment mean Children's Global Assessment Scale score was 61.4, placing the children in the 'variable functioning with sporadic difficulties or symptoms in several but not all areas' category, suggesting that these children were not severely impaired (Shaffer et al., 1983), even at treatment start. Relatedly, the investigators reported that the two children who dropped out of the study were the most severely impaired of all study participants as they both had an Anxiety Disorders Interview Schedule Clinician Severity Rating of 7 out of 8 for their primary anxiety disorder diagnosis, with 0 indicating no impairment and 8 indicating significant impairment. Additionally, the two children who dropped out had a high number of comorbid anxiety and non-anxiety diagnoses and the lowest global functioning as measured by the Children's Global Assessment Scale. Finally, as reported by the investigators, one independent evaluator who was blind to treatment related data but not to assessment time points completed all research assessments at all time points.

In summary, Parent-Child Interaction Therapy and its derivative interventions, all of which have a strong behavioral focus, show promise in the treatment of anxiety disorders in young children, but have limited empirical evidence to document their efficacy and warrant further evaluation.

4.3   Cognitive Behavior Therapy

Traditional cognitive behavior therapy (CBT) is a form of individual psychotherapy that emphasizes the interplay among thoughts, feelings, and behaviors and proposes that thoughts cause or influence feelings and behaviors. Traditional CBT focuses on helping individuals develop and implement coping strategies to identify, challenge, and change automatic and often distorted thoughts that are generated in various situations, in order to regulate feelings engendered by the cognitive distortions, which ultimately leads to the display of more adaptive behavior. Given the importance traditional CBT assigns to recognizing, challenging, and changing thought patterns, it has often been described as too complex and cognitively sophisticated to implement directly with children under the age of eight years (e.g., Kendall, Lerner, & Craighead, 1984; Shirk, 1999; Weisz & Weersing, 1999). As a result, despite the strong evidence for its efficacy in the treatment of anxiety disorders in children eight years and older (e.g., Cartwright-Hatton, Roberts, Chitsabesan, Fothergill, & Harrington, 2004; Kendall, Furr, & Podell, 2010; Walkup, Albano, Piacentini, Birmaher, Compton, Sherrill, et al., 2008), CBT has had limited clinical use (and related research) in young anxious children until recently. In fact, early CBT-based interventions for anxious children younger than eight years of age were initially delivered only to the parents and not to the children directly. For example, Rapee and colleagues used parent-focused education groups to deliver CBT to parents of behaviorally inhibited children under eight years of age (Rapee, Kennedy, Ingram, Edwards, & Sweeney, 2005; Rapee, Kennedy, Ingram, Edwards, & Sweeney, 2010), while Santacruz and colleagues taught parents how to implement exposure programs (Santacruz, Méndez, & Sánchez-Meca, 2006) and others have delivered CBT to parents of anxious young children in the format of parent-only group sessions (Cartwright-Hatton et al., 2011; Kennedy, Rapee, & Edwards, 2009). Although important early initiatives, these parent-focused treatment approaches are not directly discussed here as this chapter focuses primarily on CBT interventions delivered directly to young anxious children under eight years of age.

More recently, innovative approaches have been developed for directly involving children under eight years old in the treatment process by teaching them aspects of

CBT strategies. For example, clinical research groups have used dyadic parent-child sessions (e.g., Hirshfeld-Becker, Masek, Henin, Blakely, Rettew, Dufton, et al., 2008) while others have utilized separate and concurrently held parent groups and child groups to deliver CBT to young children (e.g., Monga, Rosenbloom, Tanha, Owens, & Young, 2015; Monga, Young, & Owens, 2009; Waters, Ford, Wharton, & Cobham, 2009). With the exception of the Taming Sneaky Fears program (Monga et al., 2009, 2015), which is described at length in Chaps. 5–11, most CBT interventions focus primarily on behavior (exposure hierarchies) and feelings in the direct work with young anxious children, with little attention paid to the cognitive distortions that are a hallmark of anxiety disorders. Examples of such interventions are described below.

4.3.1   Parent-Child Dyadic Approach

Hirshfeld-Becker and colleagues used a 20-session intervention called Being Brave: A Program for Coping with Anxiety for Young Children and Their Parents (Hirshfeld-Becker et al., 2008), which is an adaptation of the manualized Coping Cat program (Kendall, Kane, Howard, & Siqueland, 1992), originally developed for older anxious children. The Being Brave program's initial six parent-only sessions provide parents with psychoeducation about anxiety and anxiety management, parenting skills, and information on how to develop and use graded exposures with their children. The Being Brave intervention's main focus is primarily behavioral, although an effort is made to help children identify feeling states. Hirshfeld-Becker and colleagues hypothesize that graduated exposure is the primary approach to use for reducing child anxiety symptoms and so sessions 7 through 20 are dyadic parent-child sessions during which the therapist focuses on helping children understand the rationale for treatment and learn basic coping strategies, such as recognizing anxious feelings and implementing a coping plan in order to complete exposures. As such, children are introduced to the idea of working on 'being brave.' They learn relaxation strategies in session 7 and how to develop 'coping plans' in order to begin to use exposures in session 8. The bulk of the dyadic sessions (sessions 9 to 17) focus on planning, rehearsing, and implementing graduated exposures to various feared situations. In session 18, children make a final project (a short video or book) to illustrate a strategy they learned to be brave. Session 19 consists of a party or graduation to celebrate the gains made by the child. A final session 20 is for parents only and focuses on relapse prevention.

In an open trial pilot study of the Being Brave program (Hirshfeld-Becker et al., 2008), nine children (including one who did not meet criteria for an anxiety disorder at baseline) completed a mean number of 17.1 sessions ($SD = 2.4$). At post-treatment, six (66.7%) of the nine children no longer met criteria for an anxiety disorder.

In a follow-up randomized control trial using the same Being Brave program (Hirshfeld-Becker, Masek, Henin, Blakely, Pollock-Wurman, McQuade et al., 2010), 64 four- to seven-year-old children (M age = 5.4 years; $SD = 1.0$) with various anxiety disorders diagnosed using the Schedule for Affective Disorders and

Schizophrenia, Epidemiologic Version (Orvaschel, 1994) were randomized to either the dyadic parent-child CBT arm ($N = 34$) or a 6-month waitlist condition arm ($N = 30$). Seventy-seven percent of children had more than one anxiety disorder at baseline. Children in the two arms did not differ on any of the baseline measures such as demographic variables, number of comorbid diagnoses, Child Behavior Checklist (Achenbach, 1991) scores, behavioral inhibition, rates of parental anxiety, or cognitive testing using the Kaufman Brief Intelligence Test (Kaufman & Kaufman, 1990). Fifty-seven children completed the study (five dropped out and two did not attend the post-treatment assessment). Using intent-to-treat analyses, seventeen (50%) of the 34 children in the CBT arm were free of anxiety disorder post-treatment, compared to five (16.7%) of 30 children in the waitlist arm, $\chi^2(1, N = 64) = 7.85$, $p < 0.01$. At post-treatment, children in the CBT arm had a greater mean decrease in the number of anxiety diagnoses ($M = 1.72$; $SD = 1.53$), compared to children in the waitlist arm ($M = 0.93$; $SD = 1.30$), $z = -2.21$, $p < 0.05$. Additionally, significantly better Clinical Global Impression—Improvement (Guy & Bonato, 1970) scores were seen for children with social anxiety ($t = -3.04$; $p < 0.01$), separation anxiety disorder ($t = -2.12$, $p < 0.05$), and specific phobia ($t = -2.20$, $p < 0.05$), while no significant improvement was reported in children with generalized anxiety disorder ($t = -0.090$, p = n.s.) and agarophobia ($t = -0.057, p$ = n.s.).

At one-year follow-up, seven (24%) of the 29 children who had completed the dyadic CBT program had sought out further treatment. Of the 22 children who had not had further treatment, 15 (68%) were free of anxiety diagnosis. The authors did not provide additional information to explain why nearly a quarter of children who participated in the dyadic CBT program sought out further treatment.

Results from this randomized control trial show support for the use of graduated exposures in the treatment of various anxiety disorders in young children.

4.3.2 Child Group Approaches

In this section, we describe the Take ACTION program, a group CBT protocol developed by Waters and colleagues (Waters, Donaldson, & Zimmer-Gembeck, 2008; Waters, Wharton, Zimmer-Gembeck, & Craske, 2008; Waters et al., 2009) and an open trial of the Fun FRIENDS program with preschoolers (Barrett, Fisak, & Cooper, 2015). As previously mentioned, another evidence-based group CBT program for the treatment of anxiety disorders in young children, Taming Sneaky Fears (Monga et al., 2009, 2015), is described in detail in Chaps. 5–11.

4.3.2.1 Take Action Program

The Take ACTION program (Waters, Donaldson, et al., 2008; Waters, Wharton, et al., 2008; Waters et al., 2009) is a ten-week manualized program developed for children between ages four and 18 years. It includes a child component and a parent component. The child program uses modules around the acronym 'Take ACTION' that include: 'be AWARE' of anxiety and body reactions to anxiety; 'keep CALM' and learn relaxation techniques; 'THINK strong thoughts' as a reminder to identify anxious self-talk and use coping statements and calm thoughts instead; 'INITIATE action' when faced with graded exposures; 'use my OPTIONS' as a reminder for children to use the strength cards they develop and problem solving skills, and identify a strong team (e.g., others who support them); and 'NEVER stop taking action' as a reminder to develop confident nonverbal behavior, including being assertive when dealing with bullies.

In a randomized control trial using the Take ACTION program (Waters et al., 2009), 80 four- to eight-year-old children who met criteria for an anxiety disorder using the Anxiety Disorders Interview Schedule (Silverman & Albano, 1996) and their parents were randomized to one of three treatment arms: a Parent + Child CBT group arm ($N = 31$; M age = 6.89 years; $SD = 1.25$), a Parent Only CBT group arm ($N = 38$; M age = 6.68 years; $SD = 1.2$), or a waitlist control arm ($N = 11$; M age = 6.79 years; $SD = 1.03$). Parents in the Parent + Child CBT group arm and the Parent Only CBT group arm received the same content. Children in the Parent + Child CBT group arm attended ten one-hour, weekly group sessions with a therapist and received a workbook containing the weekly sessions' curriculum. Children in the Parent Only CBT group arm did not attend any group program; instead, each week while at the parent session, their parents received the relevant section of the children's workbook to work on at home with their children during the week.

There were no statistically significant differences among groups at baseline on demographic variables, primary anxiety disorder severity ratings, number of comorbid diagnoses, or any other measures (Waters et al., 2009). Five children withdrew prior to randomization. Post-treatment assessments using the Anxiety Disorders Interview Schedule were completed by one of the group therapists; however, the six- and 12-month follow-up assessments were conducted by independent raters, blind to children's diagnostic status and treatment condition. At post-treatment, using intent-to-treat analyses, 18.2% of children in the waitlist control, 54.8% of children in the Parent + Child CBT group arm, and 55.3% of children in the Parent Only CBT group arm no longer met criteria for a primary anxiety disorder. Compared to children in the waitlist control arm, the number of children who no longer met criteria for their primary anxiety disorder was significantly greater in the Parent + Child CBT group arm, χ^2 (1, $N = 41$) = 4.79 $p < 0.05$, and in the Parent-Only CBT group arm, χ^2 (1, $N = 49$) = 4.71, $p < 0.05$. There were, however, no significant differences at post-treatment between the two treatment arms, χ^2 (1, $N = 68$) = 0.01, p = n.s.

Six months post-treatment, using intent-to-treat analyses, no statistical differences were noted between the two treatment arms with respect to loss of primary anxiety diagnosis, with 55% of children in the Parent + Child CBT group arm and 58% of children in the Parent Only CBT group arm no longer meeting criteria for their primary anxiety disorder diagnosis, χ^2 (1, $N = 69$) = 0.07, p = n.s. Similar findings were reported 12 months post-treatment, with 55% of children in each treatment arm no longer meeting criteria for their primary anxiety disorder diagnosis, χ^2 (1, $N = 69$) = 0.03, p = n.s. Although not statistically significant, higher dropout rates were reported in the Parent Only CBT group arm (26% or ten of 38 children), compared to the Parent + Child CBT group arm (16% or five of 31 children), $\chi^2 (1, N = 20) = 0.70, p = $ n.s.

The Waters and colleagues (2009) study is one of the first studies on the treatment of anxiety disorders in young children that used a randomized control design to compare two active treatments and a waitlist control group with young anxious children. Waters and colleagues (2009) note that their study may not have been adequately powered to detect statistically significant results between the two treatment arms and that this may have contributed to the lack of differences noted. They further suggest that parents in the Parent + Child CBT group arm may have expected therapists in the children's group to provide all the necessary instruction to children and therefore may not have practiced and/or supported their children as much as expected between sessions, thus contributing to the lack of difference between treatments. This observation highlights the pivotal role that parents play in the treatment of anxious young children. Additionally, although the investigators did not highlight this, it is possible that the approach and terminology used in the Take ACTION program, developed for a broader age range, may not have been as developmentally appropriate for the younger four- to eight-year-old age group in the study sample. If accurate, this observation would highlight the importance of engaging younger children at their developmental level.

4.3.2.2 Fun FRIENDS Program

The Fun FRIENDS group CBT program was developed specifically for five- to seven-year-old children and is an offshoot of the FRIENDS for Life program, a social skills and resilience building program that is recognized by the World Heath Organization as an effective program to prevent anxiety in children aged eight to 11 (Barrett, 2007a, 2007b). The Fun Friends group CBT program is primarily a child-based group intervention with children attending ten weekly, 90-minute group sessions with therapists who meet separately with the parents for the last 20 minutes of each session to inform parents about the skills their children learned during the child group session and how to use appropriate reinforcement at home (Barrett, 2007a, 2007b). Additionally, parents attend two parent information sessions as part of the treatment program. The child program outline follows the acronym 'FRIENDS,' with the first session devoted to introducing participants to the group and presenting the concept of 'being brave.' Sessions 2 and 3 focus on the 'F' for feeling recognition, followed by coping with feelings through 'thumbs-up' (helpful) and 'thumbs-down' (unhelpful) behaviors, as well as recognizing the link between feelings and behavior. Session 4 teaches 'R' for relaxation and consists of teaching children various relaxation strategies. Sessions 5 and 6 focus on the 'I,' which stands for 'I can try my best' and uses a traffic light analogy with 'red' being unhelpful thoughts and 'green' being helpful thoughts, including the concept of challenging 'red' or unhelpful thoughts and finding more 'green' or helpful thoughts as a way of achieving goals. Session 7 uses the 'E' for Encourage as a way of trying new things by breaking them into smaller steps and using 'green' thoughts to help achieve goals. Session 8 is 'N' for Nurture and brings in the idea of role models and support teams as people who help with achieving goals. Session 9 is 'D' for 'Don't forget to be brave' and further discusses the concepts of support teams and planning ahead for difficult situations. Finally, session 10 is 'S' for 'Stay smiling' and children dress up as their favorite brave person and celebrate their success in completing the program.

Although two previous published studies have evaluated the Fun FRIENDS program as a universal prevention program (Anticich, Barrett, Silverman, Lacherez, & Gillies, 2013; Pahl & Barrett, 2010), there has been only one open treatment trial (Barrett, Fisak, & Cooper, 2015) in young children with 31 parents and children (M age = 5.68 years; SD = 0.54; range = 5–7) diagnosed with at least one anxiety disorder using the Anxiety Disorders Interview Schedule (Silverman & Albano, 1996). Barrett, Fisak, and Cooper (2015) reported that the young children who completed the Fun FRIENDS had fewer mean number of anxiety diagnoses post-treatment compared to pre-treatment, t (29) = 3.80, p < 0.01. However, the authors did not report on the type of anxiety diagnoses at pre- or post-treatment or clinical severity of the anxiety disorders. Additionally, although the authors reported a significant decrease in the total score of the Preschool Anxiety Scale (Spence, Rapee, McDonald, & Ingram, 2001) from pre-treatment to post-treatment, t (29) = 5.14, p < 0.01, they did not report the actual pre- and post-treatment data. Furthermore, as noted by the authors, attrition in the sample over the follow-up period limited the evaluation of 12-month follow-up data.

Early research with the Fun FRIENDS group CBT program shows promise. Further research is needed to evaluate this program in the treatment of young children with anxiety disorders using larger sample sizes and more rigorous methodology.

4.4 Management of Selective Mutism

Despite the fact that more than 90 reports on the treatment of selective mutism are found in the literature, the majority of these are single case reports (e.g., Cohan, Chavira, & Stein, 2006; Viana, Beidel, & Rabian, 2009). In fact, only two studies to date have used a randomized control design and these trials are described below.

4.4.1 Defocused Communication

Defocused communication is the cornerstone of a treatment program developed by Oerbeck, Johansen, Lundahl, and Kristensen (2012). Defocused communication promotes interaction with children while removing the focus from communication (e.g., sitting beside rather than facing the child, completing an activity the child enjoys, 'thinking aloud' rather than asking the child direct questions, and giving the child time to respond rather than talking for the child).

In an early pilot study, Oerbeck et al. (2012) utilized a treatment program that the authors described as CBT. It included parent psychoeducation and an individual treatment protocol of defocused communication with seven three- to five-year-old children (M age $= 52$ months; $SD = 9$) who were diagnosed with selective mutism using the Anxiety Disorders Interview Schedule (Silverman & Albano, 1996). None of the children were speaking to adults at school at the treatment start, although some spoke with peers during play activities. The two main components of this manualized program, which extended over six months, were defocused communication and behavioral intervention that included the use of rewards. The first three weekly, one-hour sessions took place in the children's home and focused on getting to know the children, developing the goals of treatment, and providing psychoeducation to parents about selective mutism and defocused communication. The following 18 sessions took place twice per week at the preschool/school for 30 minutes each time. Six speaking levels (1–6) were developed, including $1 =$ speaking to the therapist in the presence of the parent, $2 =$ speaking to the therapist without the parent being present, $3 =$ speaking to one teacher with the therapist being present, $4 =$ speaking to teachers and children with therapist present, $5 =$ speaking to teachers and children in some settings without the therapist being present, and $6 =$ speaking to teachers and children in all settings without the therapist being present (i.e., no different than other same-aged peers).

Results from the early pilot study show improvement in speaking behaviors and in teacher reports of selective mutism symptoms at post-treatment, with six (86%) of the seven children speaking in all kindergarten settings while one of the children (who also had a neurodevelopment delay) was speaking only in some kindergarten settings as assessed by the therapist working with the child and the teacher (Oerbeck et al., 2012). Although children were speaking in the kindergarten, less improvement was noted with respect to speaking in public (e.g., with strangers in the home, to the dentist, in restaurants).

This pilot study was followed by a randomized control trial (Oerbeck, Stein, Wentzel-Larsen, Langsrud, & Kristensen, 2014) with 24 three- to nine-year-old children with selective mutism (M age $= 6.5$ years, $SD = 2.0$; 8 boys). Nine (37.5%) of the 24 study children were preschoolers (three to five years of age at study start), while the remaining 13 children were older. Diagnoses were established with the parent Anxiety Disorders Interview Schedule (Silverman & Albano, 1996). All 24 children had comorbid social anxiety disorder. Fifteen (62.5%) of 24 mothers reported that their children had delays in motor or language development. Children were randomized to what the authors described as the manualized CBT treatment arm or a three-month waitlist control arm. The same protocol used in the pilot study was used in this randomized control trial. Using the School Speech Questionnaire (Bergman, Keller, Wood, Piacentini, & McCracken, 2001), a significant increase in speaking behavior was observed in the treatment arm from pre-treatment ($M = 0.68$) to post-treatment ($M = 1.22$), (0.54, 95% CI 0.19–0.89, $T_{22} = 3.22$, $p = 0.004$). No significant changes on the School Speech Questionnaire were reported in the waitlist control arm from baseline ($M = 0.44$) to three months later ($M = 0.40$), $T_{22} = -0.08$, $p = $ n.s. Of interest, using 6.5 years as a reference, a significant time by age interaction in the treatment arm was noted, $Fs_{1,21} = 5.47$, $p < 0.05$, suggesting a greater increase in speech for younger versus older children post-treatment. Although all children in the treatment arm were speaking to the therapist without the parent being present in the preschool/school setting (level 2), only three children (all of whom were preschoolers) were speaking to the teachers and children in some settings without the therapist present (level 5) by the end of treatment.

Children in the 3-month waitlist control then went on to receive treatment. Twelve months after treatment completion all 24 children were assessed (Oerbeck, Stein, Pripp, & Kristensen, 2015), at which time 12 (50%) of the 24 children no longer met diagnostic criteria for selective mutism as they spoke freely at school and five of these 12 children also no longer met criteria for social anxiety disorder. The remaining 12 (50% of the 24 children) continued to meet criteria for both selective mutism and social anxiety disorder, although four children spoke freely in some but not all settings at school and to some but not all adults. Oerbeck and colleagues highlight the importance of early intervention, based upon the better treatment response in younger children, as seven (78%) of the nine preschool (three to five years old) participants no longer met criteria for selective mutism at the 12-month follow-up, while only five (33%) of 15 children in the older six- to nine-year-old age group no longer met criteria for selective mutism.

4.4.2   Integrated Behavior Therapy for Selective Mutism

Integrated Behavior Therapy for Selective Mutism is a behavioral intervention developed specifically for young children with selective mutism (Bergman, Gonzalez, Piacentini, & Keller, 2013). It consists of 20 individual sessions with the child that take place over a 24-week period. The three initial sessions (sessions 1 to 3) focus on explaining the intervention to the child, developing rapport with the child (e.g., playing non-verbal games), and showing the child ways to assess and communicate anxiety levels. In sessions 4 to 14, therapist, parent, and child work together to implement behavioral exposure exercises within the session and plan for out-of-session exposures. Attempts at exposures are consistently reinforced and when appropriate, selected cognitive restructuring principles are used, such as having the child use coping self-statements when feeling anxious or fearful. The goals of sessions 15 to 20 are to transfer control from therapist to parent and to discuss relapse prevention, with the last two sessions (sessions 19 and 20) occurring two weeks apart, thus extending the time period of the program to 24 weeks.

Using Integrated Behavior Therapy for Selective Mutism, Bergman et al. (2013) completed a randomized control trial with 21 four- to eight-year-old (M age = 5.43 years; $SD = 1.16$; range = 4–8) children with selective mutism, as diagnosed with the parent Anxiety Disorders Interview Schedule (Silverman & Albano, 1996). Eighteen (85.7%) of 21 children had both selective mutism and social anxiety disorder. Children were randomized to either the 24-week ($N = 12$) Integrated Behavior Therapy for Selective Mutism arm or a 12-week waitlist control ($N = 9$).

No significant differences were noted at baseline between the two arms on all demographic measures or clinical characteristics. Fourteen (67%) of the 21 children who completed the 24-week Integrated Behavior Therapy for Selective Mutism program no longer met criteria for selective mutism, while no improvements in speaking behaviors were observed in the 12-week waitlist control group, $\chi^2(1) = 9.69$, $p = 0.002$. A significantly higher response rate was seen in the Integrated Behavior Therapy for Selective Mutism arm at week 24 (75% vs. 0% in the waitlist control group at week 12), $\chi^2(1) = 11.81$, $p = 0.001$, as defined by receiving a rating of 1 (very much improved) or 2 (much improved) by an independent rater blind to treatment condition on the Clinical Global Impression—Improvement scale (Guy & Bonato, 1970). Additionally, significant increases in the Selective Mutism Questionnaire (Bergman, Keller, Piacentini, & Bergman, 2008) ratings were reported in the Integrated Behavior Therapy for Selective Mutism group from baseline ($M = 0.79$; $SD = 0.36$) to week 24 ($M = 1.74$; $SD = 0.54$), $F1, 11 = 31.08$, $p < 0.001$, $\eta^2_{partial} = 0.74$, while non-significant changes were noted in the waitlist control group, $F1, 8 = 0.005$, $p =$ n.s., $\eta^2_{partial} = 0.001$. Of note, although teachers reported significant improvements in speaking behaviors in children in the treatment group on the School Speech Questionnaire (Bergman et al., 2001), they did not report significant changes in social anxiety symptoms as measured by the Social Anxiety Scale for Children Revised Teacher Version (La Greca & Stone, 1993).

4.5 Summary of Interventions for Young Anxious Children

Parent-Child Interaction Therapy and its derivative interventions and various CBT-focused interventions have used a variety of techniques such as exposure hierarchies, behavioral strategies, relaxation, psychoeducation, and other strategies to treat preschool children with various anxiety disorders. Some of these interventions show promise and all require more empirical evidence to document their efficacy and effectiveness. Studies using the approaches described by Oerbeck and colleagues (2012, 2014, 2015) and Bergman and colleagues (2013) provide preliminary support for the use of various behavioral strategies in the treatment of selective mutism, with or without social anxiety disorder. Both of these approaches for selective mutism incorporate parent psychoeducation, some degree of identification and management of emotions, and various behavioral strategies, including the development and implementation of hierarchies of gradual exposure or progressive desensitization to promote speech in young mute and socially anxious children. These components are included in the Taming Sneaky Fears program, a group CBT treatment program for anxious four- to seven-year-old children that our group developed independently from the aforementioned interventions. As seen in Chaps. 5–11, one aspect of the Taming Sneaky Fears program that makes it unique among other CBT-based interventions with children under age eight years is that it directly tackles cognitive distortions, a central tenet of CBT interventions. The Taming Sneaky Fears program is detailed in Chaps. 5–11.

References

Achenbach, T. M. (1991). *Manual for the child behavior checklist/4-18 and 1991 profile*. Burlington, VT: Department of Psychiatry, University of Vermont.

Anticich, S. J., Barrett, P. M., Silverman, W., Lacherez, P., & Gillies, R. (2013). The prevention of childhood anxiety and promotion of resilience among preschool aged children: A universal school based trial. *Advances in School Mental Health Promotion, 6,* 93–121.

Barrett, P. M. (2007a). *Fun Friends. The teaching and training manual for group leaders*. Brisbane, Australia: Fun Friends Publishing.

Barrett, P. M. (2007b). *Fun Friends. Family learning adventure: Resilience building activities for 4-, 5-, and 6-year-old children*. Brisbane, Australia: Fun Friends Publishing.

Barrett, P. M., Fisak, B., & Cooper, M. (2015). The treatment of anxiety in young children: Results of an open trial of the Fun FRIENDS program. *Behaviour Change, 32*(4), 231–242.

Bergman, R. L., Gonzalez, A., Piacentini, J., & Keller, M. L. (2013). Integrated behavior therapy for selective mutism: A randomized controlled trial pilot study. *Behaviour Research and Therapy, 51*(10), 680–689.

Bergman, R. L., Keller, M. L., Piacentini, J., & Bergman, A. J. (2008). The development and psychometric properties of the selective mutism questionnaire. *Journal of Clinical Child & Adolescent Psychology, 37*(2), 456–464.

Bergman, R. L., Keller, M. L., Wood, J., Piacentini, J., & McCracken, J. (2001). Selective mutism questionnaire: Development and findings. *Proceedings of the American Academy of Child & Adolescent Psychiatry Meeting, 48,* 163.

Brinkmeyer, M. Y., & Eyberg, S. M. (2003). Parent-child interaction therapy for oppositional children. In A. E. Kazdin (Ed.), *Evidence-based psychotherapies for children and adolescents* (pp. 204–223). New York: The Guildford Press.

Cartwright-Hatton, S., McNally, D., Field, A. P., Rust, S., Laskey, B., Dixon, C., …, Symes, W. (2011). A new parenting-based group intervention for young anxious children: Results of a randomized controlled trial. *Journal of the American Academy of Child and Adolescent Psychiatry, 50*(3), 242–251.

Cartwright-Hatton, S., Roberts, C., Chitsabesan, P., Fothergill, C., & Harrington, R. (2004). Systematic review of the efficacy of cognitive behaviour therapies for childhood and adolescent anxiety disorders. *British Journal of Clinical Psychology, 43,* 421–436.

Cohan, S. L., Chavira, D. A., & Stein, M. B. (2006). Practitioner review: Psychosocial interventions for children with selective mutism: A critical evaluation of the literature from 1990–2005. *Journal of Child Psychology and Psychiatry, 47,* 1085–1097.

Comer, J. S., Puliafico, A. C., Aschenbrand, S. G., McKnight, K., Robin, J. A., Goldfine, M. E., & Albano, A. M. (2012). A pilot feasibility evaluation of the CALM Program for anxiety disorders in early childhood. *Journal of Anxiety Disorders, 26*(1), 40–49. https://doi.org/10.1016/j.janxdis.2011.08.011.

Eyberg, S. M., Funderburk, B. W., Hembree-Kigin, T. L., McNeil, C. B., Querido, J. G., & Hood, K. (2001). Parent-child interaction therapy with behavior problem children: One and two year maintenance of treatment effects in the family. *Child and Family Behavior Therapy, 23,* 1–20.

Eyberg, S. M., Nelson, M. M., & Boggs, S. R. (2008). Evidence-based psychosocial treatments for children and adolescents with disruptive behavior. *Journal of Clinical Child and Adolescent Psychology, 37,* 215–237.

Guy, W., & Bonato, R. R. (Eds.). (1970). *Clinical global impressions*. Chevy Chase, MD: National Institute of Mental Health.

Hirshfeld-Becker, D. R., Masek, B., Henin, A., Blakely, L. R., Pollock-Wurman, R. A., McQuade, J., …, Biederman, J. (2010). Cognitive behavioral therapy for 4- to 7-year-old children with anxiety disorders: A randomized clinical trial. *Journal of Consulting Clinical Psychology, 78*(4), 498–510. https://doi.org/10.1037/a0019055.

Hirshfeld-Becker, D. R., Masek, B., Henin, A., Blakely, L. R., Rettew, D. C., Dufton, L., …, Biederman, J. (2008). Cognitive-behavioral intervention with young anxious children. *Harvard Review of Psychiatry, 16*, 113–125.

Hood, K., & Eyberg, S. M. (2003). Outcomes of parent-child interaction therapy: Mothers' reports on maintenance three to six years after treatment. *Journal of Clinical Child and Adolescent Psychology, 32*, 419–429.

Kaufman, A. S., & Kaufman, N. L. (1990). *Kaufman brief intelligence test*. Circle Pines, MN: American Guidance Services.

Kendall, P. C., Furr, J. M., & Podell, J. L. (2010). Child-focused treatment of anxiety. In J. R. Weisz & A. E. Kazdin (Eds.), *Evidence-based psychotherapies for children and adolescents*. New York, NY: Guildford Press.

Kendall, P. C., Kane, M., Howard, B., & Siqueland, L. (1992). *Cognitive behavioral therapy for anxious children: Therapist manual*. Ardmore, PA: Workbook.

Kendall, P. C., Lerner, R., & Craighead, W. E. (1984). Human development and intervention in childhood psychopathology. *Child Development, 55*, 71–82.

Kennedy, S. J., Rapee, R. M., & Edwards, S. L. (2009). A selective intervention program for inhibited preschool-aged children of parents with an anxiety disorder: Effects on current anxiety disorders and temperament. *Journal of the American Academy of Child and Adolescent Psychiatry, 48*, 602–609.

La Greca, A. M., & Stone, W. L., (1993). Social anxiety scale for children-revised: Factor structure and concurrent validity. *Journal of Clinical Child Psychology 22*(1), 17–27. https://doi.org/10.1207/s15374424jccp2201_2.

Monga, S., Rosenbloom, B. N., Tanha, A., Owens, M., & Young, A. (2015). Comparison of child-parent and parent-only cognitive-behavioral therapy programs for anxious children aged 5 to 7 years: Short- and long-term outcomes. *Journal of the American Academy of Child and Adolescent Psychiatry, 54*(2), 138–146. https://doi.org/10.1016/j.jaac.2014.10.008.

Monga, S., Young, A., & Owens, M. (2009). Evaluating a cognitive behavioral therapy group program for anxious five to seven year old children: A pilot study. *Depression and Anxiety, 26*(3), 243–250. https://doi.org/10.1002/da.20551.

Oerbeck, B., Johansen, J., Lundahl, K., & Kristensen, H. (2012). Selective mutism: A home-and kindergarten-based intervention in children 3–5 years: A pilot study. *Clinical Child Psychology and Psychiatry, 17*(3), 370–383.

Oerbeck, B., Stein, M. B., Pripp, A. H., & Kristensen, H. (2015). Selective mutism: Follow-up study 1 year after end of treatment. *European Child and Adolescent Psychiatry, 24*(7), 757–766.

Oerbeck, B., Stein, M. B., Wentzel-Larsen, T., Langsrud, O., & Kristensen, H. (2014). A randomized controlled trial of a home and school-based intervention for selective mutism: Defocused communication and behavioral techniques. *Child and Adolescent Mental Health, 19*, 192–198.

Orvaschel, H. (1994). *Schedule for affective disorder and schizophrenia for school-age children-epidemiologic version* (5th ed.). Fort Lauderdale, FL: Nova Southeastern University, Center for Psychological Studies.

Pahl, K. M., & Barrett, P. M. (2010). Preventing anxiety and promoting social and emotional strength in preschool children: A universal evaluation of the Fun FRIENDS program: A matched-pair trial. *Advances in School Mental Health Promotion, 3*, 14–25.

Pincus, D., Santucci, L. C., Ehrenreich, J. T., & Eyberg, S. M. (2008). The implementation of modified Parent-Child Interaction Therapy for youth with separation anxiety disorder. *Cognitive and Behavioral Practice, 15*, 118–125.

Puliafico, A. C., Comer, J. S., & Pincus, D. B. (2012). Adapting parent-child interaction therapy to treat anxiety disorders in young children. *Child and Adolescent Psychiatric Clinics of North America, 21*(3), 607–619. https://doi.org/10.1016/j.chc.2012.05.005.

Rapee, R. M., Kennedy, S., Ingram, M., Edwards, S. L., & Sweeney, L. (2005). Prevention and early intervention of anxiety disorders in inhibited preschool children. *Journal of Consulting and Clinical Psychology, 73*, 488–497.

Rapee, R. M., Kennedy, S., Ingram, M., Edwards, S. L., & Sweeney, L. (2010). Altering the trajectory of anxiety in at-risk young children. *American Journal of Psychiatry, 167,* 1518–1525.

Santacruz, I., Méndez, F. J., & Sánchez-Meca, J. (2006). Play therapy applied by parents for children with darkness phobia: Comparison of two programmes. *Child & Family Behavior Therapy, 28*(1), 19–35.

Shaffer, D., Gould, M. S., Brasic, J., Ambrosini, P., Fisher, P., Bird, H., & Aluwahlia, S. (1983). A children's global assessment scale (CGAS). *Archives of General Psychiatry, 40*(11), 1228–1231.

Shirk, S. R. (1999). Developmental therapy. In W. K. Silverman & T. H. Ollendick (Eds.), *Developmental issues in the clinical treatment of children.* Boston, MA: Allyn & Bacon.

Silverman, W. K. & Albano, A. M. (1996). *The Anxiety disorders interview schedule for children for DSM-IV: Clinician manual (Child and parent versions).*

Spence, S. H., Rapee, R., McDonald, C., & Ingram, M. (2001). The structure of anxiety in preschoolers. *Behavior Research and Therapy, 39*(11), 1293–1316.

Viana, A. G., Beidel, D. C., & Rabian, B. (2009). Selective mutism: A review and integration of the last 15 years. *Clinical Psychology Review, 29,* 57–67.

Walkup, J. T., Albano, A. M., Piacentini, J., Birmaher, B., Compton, S. N., Sherrill, J. T., …, Iyengar, S. (2008). Cognitive behavioral therapy, sertraline, or a combination in childhood anxiety. *New England Journal of Medicine, 359,* 2753–2766.

Waters, A. M., Donaldson, J., & Zimmer-Gembeck, M. J. (2008a). Cognitive behavioural therapy combined with an interpersonal skills component in the treatment of generalized anxiety disorder in adolescent females: A case series. *Behaviour Change, 25*(1), 35–43.

Waters, A. M., Ford, L. A., Wharton, T. A., & Cobham, V. E. (2009). Cognitive-behavioural therapy for young children with anxiety disorders: Comparison of a Child + Parent condition versus a Parent Only condition. *Behaviour Research and Therapy, 47*(8), 654–662. https://doi.org/10.1016/j.brat.2009.04.008.

Waters, A. M., Wharton, T. A., Zimmer-Gembeck, M. J., & Craske, M. G. (2008b). Threat-based cognitive biases in anxious children: Comparison with non-anxious children before and after cognitive-behavioural treatment. *Behaviour Research and Therapy, 46*(3), 358–374.

Weisz, J. R., & Weersing, V. R. (1999). Developmental outcome research. In W. K. Silverman & T. H. Ollendick (Eds.), *Developmental issues in the clinical treatment of children.* Boston, MA: Allyn & Bacon.

Chapter 5
The Taming Sneaky Fears Program: Development and Refinement

5.1 Creation of the Taming Sneaky Fears Program and Historical Context

5.1.1 Development of the Child Component

The impetus for creating a group Cognitive Behavior Therapy (CBT) program specifically tailored to meet the cognitive and emotional needs of young children between the ages of five[1] and seven years came in the early 2000s when it was noted that an increasingly large number of children referred to our Anxiety Clinic who met diagnostic criteria for a variety of anxiety disorders were under the age of eight years. As reviewed in Chap. 4, although at the time CBT was recognized as the best practice for the treatment of anxious children over age eight, no recognized treatment existed for anxious children under age eight and CBT was seen as too cognitively complex and sophisticated to implement directly with children under eight years of age (e.g., Kendall, Lerner, & Craighead, 1984; Shirk, 1999; Weisz & Weersing, 1999). Further, our academic department encouraged the use of group CBT programs in clinical and research activities that pertained to the treatment of anxiety disorders in older children, so Suneeta Monga, who was often asked to assess and treat anxious children under eight years old, endeavored to adapt traditional CBT used with children over age eight in ways that would meet the cognitive and developmental needs of anxious children under eight years old and could be used in a group format. The idea of Taming Sneaky Fears was sown.

In the early stages of creating the Taming Sneaky Fears program, Monga decided to use story telling as a central component of the program as stories typically engage, entertain, and even help young children understand and process cognitively abstract concepts. In fact, many preschool and kindergarten programs use story time to engage

---

[1]Later extended down to four years old.

© Springer Nature Switzerland AG 2018
S. Monga and D. Benoit, *Assessing and Treating Anxiety Disorders in Young Children*, https://doi.org/10.1007/978-3-030-04939-3_5

children and help them master abstract concepts. Monga wrote stories specifically for young children with the goal of teaching them complex concepts, like the CBT strategies that older children were learning to utilize in their group CBT sessions. Monga's early stories included engaging characters that brought to life, concretized, and simplified abstract and complex CBT concepts such as how to recognize, identify, and label anxiety and other feelings, how to use relaxation strategies to manage anxiety symptoms, how to understand and discuss cognitive distortions, and how to use cognitive coping strategies.

Monga incorporated large animal puppets, some of which personified the main story characters, as a means to further concretize complex and abstract concepts and actively engage five- to seven-year-old children during the group CBT sessions. Throughout the evolution of the Taming Sneaky Fears program, the large animal puppets have served three additional purposes as they have: (1) provided a form of exciting distraction to counteract the distress that some children might experience as their parents depart during the first child group session; (2) promoted active engagement by the children, as children are encouraged to choose a puppet at the start of each group and hold on to it when the story is read; and (3) allowed for children to possibly feel more comfortable speaking about anxiety symptoms their puppet experiences rather than talking about their own anxiety.

Monga also recognized the need for structure in each session, not only because CBT sessions are typically structured and manualized, but also because many preschool and kindergarten programs use predictable and consistent structure and routines to support children in their learning, and young children typically enjoy structure and predictability as this gives them a sense of control and mastery. To mirror what is done in many preschool and kindergarten programs, Monga divided the group sessions with the children into a Circle Time (when children sit in a circle, share activities that have taken place or are planned in between sessions, and review the concepts learned during the previous group CBT session), a Story Time (when children listen to a new story each week that engages children and illustrates a central CBT concept), a Craft Time (when children complete drawings to help process, reinforce, and complement the key concept taught during Story Time), and a Snack Time (when children share a snack to promote socialization among the children and between children and child group therapists). The structure for each group CBT session has remained consistent through the several refinements brought to the Taming Sneaky Fears program over time.

Another aspect of the program that has remained consistent over the years is the use of puppets to portray Sneaky Fears. In the Taming Sneaky Fears program, the child's anxiety, fears, or worries are externalized and given the name, 'Sneaky Fears.' A lot of thought was put into the portrayal of the Sneaky Fears' story character, the puppets used during group sessions to represent Sneaky Fears, and the timing of Sneaky Fears' first appearance in the group sessions. Monga viewed the puppets portraying Sneaky Fears popping out unexpectedly in the middle of the story as a necessary vehicle to allow children to externalize their anxiety symptoms and make anxiety concrete. Here were two sneaky, somewhat intimidating looking puppets[2] that made scary, untrue, and exaggerated statements and prevented the story's central character from doing things he wanted or needed to do, just like the anxiety, fears, and worries that prevent the children attending the group from doing things they want or need to do. The squeals of excitement from the children when Sneaky Fears make their first appearance, the continued enjoyment and excitement whenever the Sneaky Fears puppets appear in the group sessions, and the children's ability to verbalize that Sneaky Fears use Tricks to make children feel shy, nervous, and scared, suggested to Monga and her colleagues that young children enjoy and understand the concept that Sneaky Fears portrays. The name Sneaky Fears was created to both externalize anxiety and portray the unexpected way in which anxiety 'sneaks up,' interferes with what children want or need to do, and makes children feel shy, nervous, and scared.

5.1.2   Development of the Parent Component

The parent component of the Taming Sneaky Fears program began as a stand-alone program for parents of children with anxiety disorders under the age of eight years, created in the early 2000s by Mary Owens, a psychiatrist and colleague of Monga's. As noted in Chap. 4, like other centers around that time, our anxiety clinic used a parent-focused intervention to teach parents strategies to use with their anxious children rather than having young children participate directly in treatment. As such, Owens developed a 12-week, parent-only group program that included weekly 60 minute sessions that focused on providing parents with psychoeducation about anxiety, temperament, and how to manage their children's anxiety and behavioral concerns. The original, manualized parent program provided parents with guidance and training by a therapist, as well as a forum for parents of anxious children to support each other.

5.1.3   Combining Child and Parent Components

In 2002, Monga's newly created Taming Sneaky Fears child component for five- to seven-year-old children (Sect. 5.1.1) was combined with Owen's parent component (Sect. 5.1.2) to become the first 12-session, manualized Taming Sneaky Fears group CBT program. No modifications were made to Owen's 12-session parent group program and the new eight-session child group program was simply incorporated into the parent treatment protocol. Therefore, the first Taming Sneaky Fears group program consisted of four weekly, 60 minute parent-only sessions, followed by eight

---

[2]The puppets portraying Sneaky Fears have changed over time, going from a single dragon puppet in the early stages of development to two separate, annoying and rather unpleasant jackal-like puppets in the current program, to accommodate the changes brought to the story over time.

weekly, 60 minute parent group and child group sessions that ran separately but concurrently. One parent group therapist led the parent group sessions, while two child group therapists led the child group sessions. The first child group session began with parents and children participating in a ten- to 15-minute warm-up or ice-breaker activity in the child group room, followed by a separation upon completion of the ice-breaker activity. For all subsequent sessions, parent and child groups ran concurrently but separately in adjacent rooms.

5.2 Research on the Taming Sneaky Fears Program

5.2.1 First Feasibility Study

In 2002, Monga conducted the first feasibility study on the original, 12-session child and parent group CBT program for five- to seven-year-old children and their parents. As seen in Table 5.1, 14 children and their parents participated in this first feasibility study, which included children aged five to seven years. Both qualitative and quantitative data were obtained to assess the feasibility of conducting such a novel therapeutic approach. The main questions addressed in this feasibility study were whether parents and children would attend, whether children would engage with the program, and whether a notable change in the children's symptoms would be observed.

   To address the questions of whether parents and children would attend and children would engage with the program, a research assistant conducted interviews with parents immediately upon completion of the final group session. Overall, parents reported interest and motivation to attend the group sessions with their children, a greater awareness of their children's anxiety, and more confidence in managing this anxiety. Additionally, child group therapists completed a weekly checklist created for the feasibility study which asked about (1) children's engagement in the story, craft, and other group activities, (2) children's understanding of concepts, and (3) changes noted in children's symptoms. Based on these qualitative measures, the general impression of the child group therapists was that the children were engaged, understood concepts, and were keen to learn and practice strategies. Given that only one parent group therapist was involved in the parent group sessions, parent therapist feedback was not formally evaluated, but Owens, an experienced clinician, indicated that the parents appeared to find the material easy to understand, which was in keeping with the parents' feedback.

   To address the question of whether a notable change in the children's symptoms would be observed, parents completed the Screen for Child Related Emotional Disorders (Birmaher, Khetarpal, Brent, Cully, Balach, Kaufman, et al., 1997) at the first parent-only group session and again during the aforementioned feedback interview with the research assistant, conducted immediately upon completion of the 12-session program. Although no formal statistical analyses were conducted, parents reported

Table 5.1 Chronology of clinical and research endeavors characterizing the development and refinement of the Taming Sneaky Fears program

Date	Study[a]	Sample			
		N	Age in years M (SD) range	Male (%)	Caucasian (%)
2003–04	Feasibility	14	- 5–7	64.3	–
2005–07 (Monga et al., 2009)	Pilot, non-controlled Prospective, repeated measures	32	6.5 (0.7) 5–7	40.6	84.4
2010–14 (Monga et al., 2015)	Comparative Prospective, repeated measures, longitudinal	77	6.8 (0.8) 5–7	37.7	89.6
2014	Feasibility	7	- 4–7	14.3	85.7
2015–18	RCT	94	5.4(1.0) 4–7	28	46
2017	QI Part 1	35	6.1 (1.0) 4–7	54	51
	QI Part 2	22	6.1 (1.0) 4–7	55	55

QI Quality Improvement study
RCT randomized control trial
[a]Children in all studies met diagnostic criteria for various anxiety disorders, except for the 2014 feasibility study and the 2015–18 RCT that included only children with selective mutism with or without social anxiety disorder

improvements in their children's anxiety on this measure upon completion of the program compared to the start of the program. In addition to these parent reports, in the exit interviews with the research assistant, parents spontaneously reported general improvements in their children's coping abilities and overall cooperation, compliance, and general behavior; as well, they provided positive feedback about the content of both the parent and child programs and expressed satisfaction that the program provided them with tools to use with their anxious children.

Taken together, findings from this original feasibility study suggested that implementation of the child and parent components of the Taming Sneaky Fears group CBT program was feasible. The Taming Sneaky Fears program was ready for further scientific investigation with more rigorous design and methods.

Given the qualitative data obtained in the first feasibility study with the original 12-session Taming Sneaky Fears program, specifically that children were engaged in the stories and crafts, and to match more closely the number of parent and child group sessions, the original eight-week child group component was expanded by three sessions by adding two review sessions and one graduation session, although no new stories were written, for a total of 11 child group sessions (keeping only the first session as a parent-only session). The efficacy of this revised group CBT Taming Sneaky Fears program with one parent-only Introduction Session followed by 11 weekly parent and child group sessions held separately but concurrently, was tested in a pilot study.

5.2.2 Pilot Study

As seen in Table 5.1, the pilot study used a prospective, non-controlled, repeated measures design (Monga, Young, & Owens, 2009) and included 32 children (13 boys; M age $= 6.5$ years; $SD = 0.7$; range 5–7). The children met criteria for various anxiety disorders, diagnosed using the Anxiety Disorders Interview Schedule parent interview (Silverman & Albano, 1996). High comorbidity among the anxiety disorders was noted as 62.5% of children had two or more anxiety disorder diagnoses. Parents attended a pre-treatment assessment appointment within two weeks prior to the start of treatment and a post-treatment assessment appointment within two weeks after completion of treatment. At both time points, parents were interviewed using the Anxiety Disorders Interview Schedule parent interview and completed the Screen for Child Anxiety Related Emotional Disorders parent questionnaire (Birmaher et al., 1997) and the Revised Conners' Parent Rating Scale: Long Version (Conners, Sitarenios, Parker, & Epstein, 1998). The clinicians completing the Anxiety Disorders Interview Schedule at the two time points were not blinded to pre- and post-treatment status. However, consensus scores were used for data analyses by having experienced clinicians, blind to time of assessment and using all data generated on children independently, assign a Clinician Severity Rating on the Anxiety Disorders Interview Schedule and a global functioning rating on the Children's Global Assessment Scale (Shaffer, Gould, Brasic, Ambrosini, Fisher Bird, et al., 1983). The change in the Clinician Severity Rating of the parent interview of the Anxiety Disorders Interview Schedule was used as a primary outcome measure for this pilot study.

As reported by Monga and colleagues (2009), results of this pilot study demonstrated that the mean Anxiety Disorders Interview Schedule Clinician Severity Rating for primary anxiety diagnosis at post-treatment ($M = 3.1$, $SD = 2.3$) was significantly lower than at pre-treatment ($M = 5.6$, $SD = 0.98$), $t = 6.82$ (1,31), $p = 0.001$. Of note, a mean change of 2.0 in the Clinician Severity Rating of the Anxiety Disorders Interview Schedule is considered a significant clinical change (Bennett, Manassis, Walter, Cheung, Wilansky-Traynor, Diaz-Granados, et al., 2013). The majority (71.9%) of children with two or more anxiety diagnoses lost at least one anxiety disorder, while 43.8% no longer met criteria for any anxiety disorder. Furthermore, the Children's Global Assessment Scale, a measure of overall functioning, was used as a secondary outcome measure, with significant improvement in children's overall functioning noted at post-treatment ($M = 57.1$) compared to pre-treatment ($M = 45.9$), $t = -8.14$ (1,31), $p = 0.001$. The initial mean score of 45.9 on the Children's Global Assessment Scale indicates significant functional impairment while the change of greater than 10 points at post-treatment is seen as clinically significant (Shaffer et al., 1983).

In addition to the aforementioned clinician-rated primary and secondary outcome measures, parents completed a number of parent report questionnaires to assess for anxiety and behavioral symptom change. Although these questionnaires were not specifically developed for younger children (details in Chap. 2), they were well-validated questionnaires and were therefore used for the pilot study. As reported in Monga et al. (2009), the total score on the parent report Screen for Child Anxiety Related Emotional Disorders significantly decreased from pre- ($M = 33.8$, $SD = 13.3$) to post-treatment ($M = 25.2$, $SD = 12.5$), $t = 3.76$ (1, 28), $p = 0.001$. Mean parent scores decreased from pre-treatment to post-treatment on four of the five subscales of the Screen for Child Anxiety Related Emotional Disorders: generalized anxiety subscale (M pre-treatment $= 9.8$; $SD = 4.5$ vs. M post-treatment $= 7.5$; $SD = 3.9$), $t = 3.87$ (1,28), $p = 0.001$; separation anxiety subscale (M pre-treatment $= 7.0$; $SD = 4.1$ vs. M post-treatment $= 5.1$; $SD = 3.9$), $t = 3.09$ (1,28) $p = 0.005$; social anxiety subscale (M pre-treatment $= 10.4$; $SD = 3.4$ vs. M post-treatment $= 7.9$; $SD = 4.5$), $t = 3.51$ (1,28), $p = 0.002$; and school refusal subscale (M pre-treatment $= 2.9$; $SD = 2.4$ vs. M post-treatment $= 1.7$; $SD = 1.9$), $t = 4.35$ (1,28) $p = 0.01$. The only subscale that did not change with treatment was the panic subscale (M pre-treatment $= 3.7$; $SD = 3.8$ vs. M post-treatment $= 3.1$; $SD = 3.4$), $t = 0.75$ (1,28), $p = $ n.s., possibly because panic disorder is not a common diagnosis presenting in young children, as discussed in Chap. 1. Additionally, parent scores on the anxious/shy subscale of the Revised Conners' Parent Rating Scale: Long Version declined significantly from pre-treatment to post-treatment; however, no significant changes were noted in the psychosomatic or oppositional subscales (Monga et al., 2009).

During the course of this pilot study, a small sub-group of the sample ($N = 11$; 3 males) had to wait for treatment for a mean wait time of three months due to unavoidable closure of the clinic before they attended the group treatment. This sub-group demonstrated no change in Children's Global Assessment Scale score over this wait period; however, the post-treatment score was significantly improved ($M = 61.2$, $SD = 10.3$), $F(1,10) = 30.94$, $p < 0.001$, thus suggesting that improvement was due to treatment rather than time.

Remission rates (66.7%) for children with only one anxiety disorder were comparable to rates seen in CBT studies with older children where remission rates of 56.5% are reported (Cartwright-Hatton, Roberts, Chitsabesan, Fothergill, & Harrington, 2004). Children with two or more anxiety disorders had lower remission rates at 30%.

Results from this pilot study provided early and promising evidence for the efficacy of the revised, Introduction plus 11-session Taming Sneaky Fears group CBT program in treating five- to seven-year-old children with various anxiety disorders.

5.2.3 Comparative Study

After publication of the results of the aforementioned pilot study on the Taming Sneaky Fears group CBT program (Monga et al., 2009), Monga and her colleagues examined the question of whether the child component of the Taming Sneaky Fears program along with the parent component provided added benefit as compared to delivering the parent component alone. To address this question, Monga and her colleagues (Monga, Rosenbloom, Tanha, Owens, & Young, 2015) conducted a clinical trial that compared a Child-Parent arm (where children and their parents attended the group CBT program and received the child and parent components of the Taming Sneaky Fears program) and a Parent-Only arm (where only the parents received the parent component of the Taming Sneaky Fears program and were taught CBT skills to use with their children). In order to control for the nonspecific aspects of child group attendance, the children in the Parent-Only arm attended a weekly non-CBT group program that matched the format and duration of the Taming Sneaky Fears child sessions; however, children listened to neutral stories, played games, and completed neutral crafts while socializing with other children but did not learn any CBT concepts or skills.

As seen in Table 5.1 and as reported in Monga et al. (2015), the comparative study used a prospective, repeated-measures, comparative, longitudinal design. A total of 77 five- to seven-year-old children (M age = 6.8 years; SD = 0.8; 29 males) and their parents participated. After an initial assessment was completed and informed consent to study participation was obtained, children waited for three months during which time no treatment took place. Children and parents were not randomly assigned to intervention type; instead, the intervention format (i.e., Child-Parent or Parent-Only) was randomly assigned two weeks before the start of each treatment group. In total, eight Child-Parent and six Parent-Only groups were conducted. Forty-five five- to seven-year-old children (M age = 6.6 years; SD = 0.6; 16 males) participated in the Child-Parent arm and 32 children (M age = 7.0 years; SD = 0.8; 13 males) and their parents participated in the Parent-Only arm. Research assessments took place at five time points, including at baseline, pre-treatment (within two weeks before treatment began), post-treatment (within two weeks of treatment ending), at six months post-treatment, and at 12 months post-treatment. Initial or baseline assessments took place three months prior to the start of the group intervention.

The Clinician Severity Rating of the Anxiety Disorders Interview Schedule parent interview (Silverman & Albano, 1996) was the primary outcome measure. A secondary outcome measure was the clinician rating of the children's level of global functioning using the Children's Global Assessment Scale (Shaffer et al., 1983). Parents also completed a number of parent report measures including the Screen for Child Anxiety Related Emotional Disorders (Birmaher et al., 1997) to measure child anxiety and the Beck Anxiety Inventory (Beck & Steer, 1990) to measure self-report levels of parent anxiety.

There were no significant differences in age, gender, ethnicity, Clinician Severity Rating of primary anxiety diagnosis, clinician rating of global functioning, parent report of child symptom scores, child temperament, or self-reported parent anxiety between the two treatment arms at baseline. There were no significant changes in either treatment arm on all clinical measures between baseline and pre-group assessment three months later, indicating that no change took place without treatment. Below, we report only on results related to the post-treatment and 12-month post-treatment time points (for additional details, see Monga et al., 2015).

5.2.3.1 Results at Post-treatment

At post-treatment, significantly more children no longer met criteria for their primary anxiety disorder in the Child-Parent arm (48.9%) compared to the Parent-Only arm (12.5%) (Fischer's exact test, $p = 0.001$).

Furthermore, significant improvement, as measured by mean change in Clinician Severity Rating on the Anxiety Disorders Interview Schedule from pre- to post-treatment was noted within both treatment arms (Child-Parent arm mean change = -2.3; 95% CI = $-2.7, -1.9, p < 0.0001$ and Parent-Only arm mean change = -0.9; 95% CI = $-1.4, -0.4, p = 0.001$). More importantly, there was a significant difference between the two treatments, with the Child-Parent arm having significantly lower Clinician Severity Rating of anxiety compared to the Parent-Only arm (mean change = -1.4; 95% CI = $-2.0, -0.7, p < 0.0001$). In summary, significantly greater reductions in anxiety disorder severity were seen in the Child-Parent arm as compared to the Parent-Only arm, thus providing evidence for the added benefit the child group sessions confer to the Taming Sneaky Fears group CBT program.

Global functioning of children, as measured by mean change in Children's Global Assessment Scale improved in both treatment arms (Child-Parent arm mean change = 10.3; 95% CI = 8.7, 11.9, $p < 0.0001$ and Parent-Only arm mean change = 2.5; 95% CI = 0.6, 4.5, $p = 0.01$). Again there was significantly greater improvement in global functioning in the Child-Parent arm as compared with the Parent-Only arm (mean change = 7.8; 95% CI = 5.3, 10.3, $p < 0.0001$), thus providing support for the added benefits the child group sessions confer to the Taming Sneaky Fears program.

Improvements in parent report of anxiety symptoms, as measured by changes in the total score of the parent Screen for Child Anxiety Related Emotional Disorders (mean change = $-5.6 (-9.1, -2.2) p = 0.002$), were seen in the Child-Parent arm while only significant changes in the separation anxiety factor of the parent Screen for Child Anxiety Related Emotional Disorders (mean change = $-1.6 (-2.6, -0.6)$, $p = 0.002$) were noted in the Parent-Only arm. The observation that in the Parent-Only arm parent-reported improvements were only noted in the separation anxiety subscale of the Screen for Child Anxiety Related Emotional Disorders may have been related to the fact that even in the Parent-Only arm, parents and children had learned to separate for parent and child group attendance.

5.2.3.2 Results at 12 Months Post-treatment

At 12 months post-treatment, 77.8% of children no longer met criteria for a primary anxiety diagnosis in the Child-Parent arm, while 37.5% did not meet criteria for a primary anxiety diagnosis in the Parent-Only arm. Again, significant reductions in Anxiety Disorders Interview Schedule Clinician Severity Rating were seen in both treatment arms (mean change of -3.3, 95% CI = $-3.8, -2.9, p < 0.0001$ in the Child-Parent arm and a mean change of -1.9, 95% CI = $-2.6, -1.3, p < 0.0001$ in the Parent-Only arm), with a greater improvement observed in the Child-Parent arm as compared to Parent-Only arm (mean change $= -1.4, 95\%$ CI $= -2.2, -0.6\ p =$ 0.001).

Global functioning, as measured by the Children's Global Assessment Scale, improved significantly in both treatment arms (Child-Parent arm mean change was 19.0, 95% CI $= 16.5, 21.5, p < 0.0001$, while in the Parent-Only arm mean change was 7.0, 95% CI $= 3.8, 10.2, p < 0.0001$), but again, the children in the Child-Parent arm were functioning significantly better (mean change $= 12.0\ 95\%$ CI $= 7.9, 16.0, p < 0.0001$) than the children in the Parent-Only arm.

Parent total scores on the Screen for Child Anxiety Related Emotional Disorders were again significantly reduced (mean change $= -8.3\ (-12.1, -4.4)\ p < 0.0001$) in the Child-Parent arm; as well, significant improvements on several subscales were noted: separation anxiety subscale (mean change $= -1.8\ (-2.7, -0.8), p = 0.001$), social anxiety subscale (mean change $= -2.1, (-3.2, -1.1), p = 0.0002$), and school refusal subscale (mean change $= -1.0, p = 0.002$). In the Parent-Only arm, significant improvements were again noted in the separation anxiety subscale (mean change $= -2.9\ (-4.2, -1.6), p < 0.0001$) and in the total score of the Screen for Child Anxiety Related Emotional Disorders (mean change $= -9.4\ (-14.4, -4.4)\ p = 0.0004$).

5.2.3.3   Summary of Comparative Study

Results of this comparative study suggest that without treatment, anxiety disorders in young children may not improve, given that there were no changes during the three-month no-treatment wait time. Numerous changes were noted as a result of treatment, and results suggest that treatment, not time, accounted for these changes. Study results further suggest that providing both the child and parent components of the Taming Sneaky Fears program is more efficacious in decreasing the children's severity of anxiety diagnoses and improving the children's overall functioning than providing only the parent component. Additionally, the results from the comparative study provide empirical evidence that five- to seven-year-old children can learn and utilize CBT strategies when taught in an age-appropriate, fun, and playful fashion.

5.2.3.4   Selective Mutism and Social Anxiety Disorder Data

Data from a subgroup of 24 children who participated in the Child-Parent arm of the comparative study (Monga et al., 2015) and had a primary diagnosis of either selective mutism or social anxiety disorder, were re-examined. Thirty-eight percent of these children no longer met criteria for either diagnosis post-treatment and 71% no longer met criteria for either diagnosis at 12 months post-treatment. These findings provided early evidence for the efficacy of the Taming Sneaky Fears program in the treatment of selective mutism and/or social anxiety disorder in five- to seven-year-old children. These findings also provided the impetus for the next research endeavor as despite these encouraging findings, clinical experience with young children with selective mutism and social anxiety disorder suggested that the Taming Sneaky Fears program could be further refined to specifically target symptoms of selective mutism and social anxiety disorder.

5.2.4 Selective Mutism and Social Anxiety Disorder Feasibility Study

As seen in Table 5.1, in 2014, Monga and Benoit ran a feasibility study with four- to seven-year-old children with selective mutism and/or social anxiety disorder and their parents, using a slightly revised version of the Taming Sneaky Fears program than had been used for the comparative study. These changes included: (1) the inclusion of children as young as four years old; (2) the use of specific progressive desensitization or gradual exposure strategies in both the parent and child components of the program, referred to as Climbing Bravery Ladders; (3) an expanded emphasis on psychoeducation about selective mutism and social anxiety disorder and progressive desensitization or gradual exposure strategies in the parent component; and (4) a reduction in the total number of sessions from 12 to ten (one Introduction Session with parents only, followed by nine child and parent group sessions held separately but concurrently).

The purpose of the feasibility study was threefold: (1) test the hypothesis that an emphasis on gradual exposure or progressive desensitization (or Climbing Bravery Ladders) in the parent and child components was a viable and useful tool to treat young selectively mute and socially anxious children; (2) determine the feasibility of implementing the revised program with children as young as four years old; and (3) use the data from the feasibility study to develop a larger, randomized control trial to assess the efficacy of the revised ten-session Taming Sneaky Fears program in treating four- to seven-year-old children with selective mutism with or without social anxiety disorder. This feasibility study included seven four- to seven-year-old children (1 male) with selective mutism with or without social anxiety disorder. The (qualitative) feasibility study suggested that the revisions were well received as therapists noted, and parents verbally reported, improvements in children post-treatment, with only one child requiring ongoing follow-up within our clinic after completing the group program.

5.2.5 Current Randomized Control Trial

As seen in Table 5.1, we have just completed a randomized control trial that examined the efficacy of the revised ten-session Taming Sneaky Fears group CBT program, comparing it to a ten-session Parent Psychoeducation and Child Socialization (non-CBT) group program. At this time, recruitment and data collection are complete and we are in the midst of data analyses so final results are still pending. We describe herein details about the study protocol.

Upon obtaining informed consent, subjects were randomized to either (1) the Taming Sneaky Fears parent and child CBT group program that contained the revisions for selective mutism and social anxiety disorder as described in the aforementioned feasibility study (Sect. 5.2.4) or (2) the Parent Psychoeducation and Child Socialization comparison (non-CBT) group program. Both programs were similar in duration and frequency (45 minute, weekly sessions for 11 consecutive weeks), provided children with equal opportunities for interaction and socialization with peers and group leaders, and provided parents with equal opportunities for discussion and education. In the Taming Sneaky Fears program, children and parents learned CBT concepts and strategies as described in Chaps. 6–11, while in the Parent Psychoeducation and Child Socialization program parents learned strategies for parenting and child behavior management and the children heard stories and engaged in games that focused on learning how to be friendly and how to make friends. Trained clinicians, blinded to all previous measures and treatment assignment, completed post-intervention assessments.

This randomized control trial differs from previous studies with the Taming Sneaky Fears program in that it: (1) includes children as young as four years old (to address both clinical needs and the 'natural history' of social anxiety disorder and selective mutism); (2) examines various within-the-child and within-the-parent/environment factors to determine how these relate to treatment outcome (a logistic regression analysis is planned to explore the impact of within-the-child factors such as age, gender, temperament, speech-language difficulties, and within-the-parent/environment factors such as family history of anxiety disorders, stress, immigration on treatment outcome); and (3) uses a longitudinal, repeated measures, randomized control trial, with multiple informants and a large enough sample size to give the necessary power for testing hypotheses.

Ninety-four four- to seven-year-old children (M age $= 5.44$ years: $SD = 1.0$; 28 males) with a primary diagnosis of selective mutism and/or social anxiety disorder, diagnosed using the parent interview of the Anxiety Disorders Interview Schedule (Silverman & Albano, 1996), were enrolled in this study. Assessments took place at three different time points, including baseline or pre-treatment, within two weeks of treatment ending or post-treatment, and at six months post-treatment. A speech-language assessment was conducted at baseline and a number of measures described in Chap. 2 were used, including the Preschool Anxiety Scale (Spence & Rapee, 1999), the Selective Mutism Questionnaire (Bergman, Keller, Piacentini, & Bergman, 2008), and the School Speech Questionnaire (Bergman, Keller, Wood, Piacentini, & McCracken, 2001). Additionally, a number of the newly developed tools, described in Chap. 3, were administered, including the Pre-SCARED, the Steps to Talking, the Selective Mutism versus Social Anxiety Disorder Criteria Checklist, the Talking Behavior Assessment Tool, and the Mutism Accommodation Scale.

The randomized control trial was completed in December 2017 and we are currently conducting data analyses.

5.2.6 Quality Improvement Study

While the aforementioned randomized controlled trial was being conducted, Monga and Benoit continued to refine the Taming Sneaky Fears program and evaluate the impact of changes brought to the program. One major additional refinement included the creation of an illustrated children's storybook and companion workbook, *Taming Sneaky Fears – Leo the Lion's story of bravery* & *Inside Leo's den: The workbook* (Benoit & Monga, 2018b), which has also been translated into the French language, *Apprivoiser les Peurs-pas-fines – L'histoire de bravoure de Léo le lionceau* & *Dans la tanière de Léo: Le cahier de travail* (Benoit & Monga, 2018a). The English language storybook and companion workbook are now being used as the basis to deliver the child component of the Taming Sneaky Fears program in our clinic. A second refinement included a reduction in the total number of sessions from ten to nine (one parent-only Introduction Session followed by eight child and parent group sessions held separately but concurrently; thus going back to the original number of sessions Monga had envisioned when she first developed the Taming Sneaky Fears program in the early 2000s).

The Hospital for Sick Children authorized Monga and Benoit to conduct a Quality Improvement study to obtain feedback from parents and children and evaluate the further revised version of the Taming Sneaky Fears program, as the Taming Sneaky Fears group CBT program has become the standard of care at the Hospital for Sick Children. This Quality Improvement study was completed between December 2016 and August 2017. According to the hospital policy, this work was primarily intended to improve the current standard of care and not to provide generalizable, scientific knowledge in this field, and as such it was exempt from Research Ethics Board review. Although there was no formal consenting process, permission was still obtained from parents to participate in the Quality Improvement study, which involved two parts, as described below.

As seen in Table 5.1, thirty-five four- to seven-year-old children (M age = 6.1 years; $SD = 1.0$; 19 males) and their parents participated in the first part of the Quality Improvement study in which parents were asked to rate main aspects of the revised Taming Sneaky Fears program, using a five-point rating scale, with 4 = very helpful, 3 = quite helpful, 2 = somewhat helpful, 1 = a little helpful, and 0 = not at all helpful. A mean score of 3.26 ($SD = 0.72$) was obtained for the question, 'How helpful was the Taming Sneaky Fears program to you in figuring out how to help your child?' A mean score of 3.00 ($SD = 0.84$) was obtained for the question, 'How helpful was the Taming Sneaky Fears program to your child in learning how to manage anxiety symptoms?' Parents' responses to these two main questions suggested that parents who participated in this small Quality Improvement study found the revised Taming Sneaky Fears program helpful overall.

As mentioned, the purpose of a Quality Improvement study is not to provide scientific evidence, therefore the data provided below are descriptive only, must not be viewed as empirical evidence, and require formal scientific confirmation with proper ethical approval and scientific design. A subgroup of 22 children (*M* age = 6.1 years; *SD* = 1.07; 12 males) with a primary anxiety disorder diagnosis as diagnosed using the parent interview of the Anxiety Disorders Interview Schedule (Silverman & Albano, 1996), participated in the second part of the Quality Improvement study as they attended both a baseline and post-treatment follow-up assessment visit within two weeks of group treatment initiation or completion as protocolized in our previous research studies. This Quality Improvement sample of 22 children was not significantly different from the sample of children who participated in the comparative research study described in Sect. 5.2.3 on gender, enthnicity, baseline Anxiety Disorders Interview Schedule Clinician Severity Rating, or Children's Global Assessment Scale score; however, the Quality Improvement sample was slightly older (*M* age = 6.1 years; *SD* = 1.1); as compared with the comparative research study sample (*M* age = 5.5 years; *SD* = 1.0; $t(66) = -2.1, p = 0.040$).

Of note, the two clinical assessments conducted as part of the Quality Improvement study were conducted by independent but non-blinded clinicians. Data analyses, in the context of a Quality Improvement study with its significant limitations (e.g., meant to be descriptive only and without the stringent ethical and scientific requirements of research studies), provide clinical support that the revised nine-session Taming Sneaky Fears program might be as efficacious as the previous ten-session program, based on the following: (1) baseline Anxiety Disorders Interview Schedule Clinician Severity Rating (*M* = 5.73; *SD* = 1.07) significantly decreased post-treatment (*M* = 4.5; *SD* = 2.16) $t = 3.47$ (1,21), $p = 0.002$; (2) Children's Global Assessment Scale scores improved significantly from pre-treatment (*M* = 48.3; *SD* = 10.17) to post-treatment (*M* = 57.7; SD = 15.80) $Z = -3.140, p = 0.002$; and (3) parent report on the Spence Preschool Anxiety Scale (Spence & Rapee, 1999) improved significantly from baseline 44.19 (*SD* = 18.86) to post-treatment 37.52 (*SD* = 15.65), $t = 2.60$ (1,20), $p = 0.017$. In addition, parents completed the Spence Preschool Anxiety Scale (Spence & Rapee, 1999) at baseline and post-treatment with total scores improving significantly from 44.19 (*SD* = 18.86) to 37.52 (*SD* = 15.65), $t = 2.60$ (1,20), $p = 0.017$.

The results from this Quality Improvement study provide descriptive support only, and warrant replication using scientifically sound design. However, together with clinical experience with the revised nine-session program, they provide cautious confidence that the revised (and current) nine-session Taming Sneaky Fears group CBT program continues to be helpful to young anxious children and their parents. The current Taming Sneaky Fears program is detailed in Chaps. 6–11.

References

Beck, A. T., & Steer, R. A. (1990). *Manual for the Beck anxiety inventory*. San Antonio, TX: Psychological Corporation.

Bennett, K., Manassis, K., Walter, S. D., Cheung, A., Wilansky-Traynor, P., Diaz-Granados, et al. (2013). Cognitive behavioral therapy age effects in child and adolescent anxiety: An individual patient data metaanalysis. *Depression and Anxiety, 30*(9), 829–841.

Benoit, D., & Monga, S. (2018a). *Apprivoiser les Peurs-pas-fines—L'histoire de bravoure de Léo le lionceau & Dans la tanière de Léo: Le cahier de travail*. Victoria, British Columbia: FriesenPress.

Benoit, D., & Monga, S. (2018b). *Taming sneaky fears—Part A. Leo the Lion's story of bravery and Part B. Inside Leo the Lion's den: How to tame your Sneaky Fears*. Victoria, B.C.: FriesenPress.

Bergman, R. L., Keller, M. L., Piacentini, J., & Bergman, A. J. (2008). The development and psychometric properties of the selective mutism quesitonnaire. *Journal of Clinical Child and Adolescent Psychology, 37*(2), 456–464.

Bergman, R. L., Keller, M. L., Wood, J., Piacentini, J., & McCracken, J. (2001). Selective mutism questionnaire: development and FINDINGS. *Proceedings of the American Academy of Child and Adolescent Psychiatry Meeting, 48,* 163.

Birmaher, B., Khetarpal, S., Brent, D., Cully, M., Balach, L., Kaufman, J., et al. (1997). The Screen for Child Anxiety Related Emotional Disorders (SCARED): Scale construction and psychometric characteristics. *Journal of the American Academy of Child and Adolescent Psychiatry, 36*(4), 545–553. https://doi.org/10.1097/00004583-199704000-00018.

Cartwright-Hatton, S., Roberts, C., Chitsabesan, P., Fothergill, C., & Harrington, R. (2004). Systematic review of the efficacy of cognitive behaviour therapies for childhood and adolescent anxiety disorders. *British Journal of Clinical Psychology, 43,* 421–436.

Conners, C. K., Sitarenios, G., Parker, J. D., & Epstein, J. N. (1998). The revised Conners' Parent Rating Scale (CPRS-R): Factor structure, reliability, and criterion validity. *Journal of Abnormal Child Psychology, 26*(4), 257–268.

Kendall, P. C., Lerner, R., & Craighead, W. E. (1984). Human development and intervention in childhood psychopathology. *Child Development, 55,* 71–82.

Monga, S., Rosenbloom, B. N., Tanha, A., Owens, M., & Young, A. (2015). Comparison of child-parent and parent-only cognitive-behavioral therapy programs for anxious children aged 5 to 7 years: Short- and long-term outcomes. *Journal of the American Academy of Child and Adolescent Psychiatry, 54*(2), 138–146. https://doi.org/10.1016/j.jaac.2014.10.008.

Monga, S., Young, A., & Owens, M. (2009). Evaluating a cognitive behavioral therapy group program for anxious five to seven year old children: a pilot study. *Depression and Anxiety, 26*(3), 243–250. https://doi.org/10.1002/da.20551.

Shaffer, D., Gould, M. S., Brasic, J., Ambrosini, P., Fisher, P., Bird, H., et al. (1983). A children's global assessment scale (CGAS). *Archives of General Psychiatry, 40*(11), 1228–1231.

Shirk, S. R. (1999). Developmental therapy. In W. K. Silverman & T. H. Ollendick (Eds.), *Developmental issues in the clinical treatment of children*. Boston, MA: Allyn & Bacon.

Silverman, W. K., & Albano, A. M. (1996). *The Anxiety disorders interview schedule for children for DSM-IV: Clinician manual (Child and parent versions)*.

Spence, S. H., & Rapee, R. (1999). The preschool anxiety scale. Retrieved from http://www.scaswebsite.com/docs/scas-preschool-scale.pdf.

Weisz, J. R., & Weersing, V. R. (1999). Developmental outcome research. In W. K. Silverman & T. H. Ollendick (Eds.), *Developmental issues in the clinical treatment of children*. Boston, MA: Allyn & Bacon.

Chapter 6
The Taming Sneaky Fears Program: Theoretical Framework, Requirements for Implementation, and Program Overview

6.1 Theoretical Framework

The Taming Sneaky Fears program is a unique Cognitive Behavior Therapy (CBT) group treatment program that was developed specifically for anxious four- to seven-year-old children and their parents, as described in Chap. 5. In the child group sessions, four- to seven-year-old anxious children learn complex concepts (e.g., feeling states, cognitive distortions) and sophisticated skills to enable them to manage their anxiety (e.g., relaxation techniques, cognitive coping strategies, and progressive desensitization or gradual exposure) through the use of young child-friendly terminology, a children's story and companion workbook (*Taming Sneaky Fears—Leo the Lion's story of bravery & Inside Leo's den: The workbook*[1] (Benoit & Monga, 2018a, b), created specifically for the program), puppets, games, and crafts. In the parent group sessions, parents learn the same concepts and skills, which they are urged to implement in their every day life with their young anxious children.

---

[1] *Taming Sneaky Fears—Leo the Lion's story of bravery & Inside Leo's den: The Workbook* has been translated into the French language, *Apprivoiser les Peurs-pas-fines—L'histoire de bravoure de Léo le lionceau & Dans la tanière de Léo: Le cahier de travail* (Benoit & Monga, 2018a, b). Translation into other languages is being considered.

Electronic supplementary material The online version of this chapter (https://doi.org/10.1007/978-3-030-04939-3_6) contains supplementary material, which is available to authorized users.

© Springer Nature Switzerland AG 2018
S. Monga and D. Benoit, *Assessing and Treating Anxiety Disorders in Young Children*, https://doi.org/10.1007/978-3-030-04939-3_6

6.1.1   Adapting Traditional CBT for Young Children

6.1.1.1   Psychoeducation Component of Traditional CBT

In traditional CBT for anxiety disorders, therapists provide children, adolescents, and adults with information (psychoeducation) about what anxiety is, how to recognize anxiety symptoms and triggers, and how to manage and cope with anxiety symptoms.

When working with four- to seven-year-old children, information about anxiety, anxiety symptoms, triggers, and coping strategies needs to be conveyed in a simple, concrete, and young child-friendly manner. In Taming Sneaky Fears, the abstract concept of anxiety is made concrete by *externalizing* anxiety. In other words, and as suggested by others (e.g., Huebner, 2006), young children and their parents learn to think of anxiety as an unwanted visitor that they are tired of hosting, a separate entity with its own name rather than an integral and unchangeable part of the child. Young children and parents are encouraged to give this unwanted and bothersome visitor a name so they have a common language to refer to it. In the Taming Sneaky Fears program, Sneaky Fears is the name given to this unwanted visitor.

Albeit externalized, the concept of anxiety or Sneaky Fears is still abstract for four- to seven-year-old children. So to make the abstract concept of anxiety or Sneaky Fears even more concrete, two related strategies are used. First, the illustrated children's story section of *Taming Sneaky Fears—Leo the Lion's story of bravery & Inside Leo's den: The workbook* (Benoit & Monga, 2018a, b) is used at each child session to bring to life Sneaky Fears, these two annoying jackal characters that continuously bother the main story character, Leo the Lion, by appearing throughout the story and saying worry thoughts (cognitive distortions) in a growling voice (creating fear and anxiety for Leo). Second, during the child group sessions, Sneaky Fears are portrayed by two full body, gray fox puppets that are referred to as jackals to match the children's story characters. Externalizing anxiety and making the abstract concept of anxiety concrete and come to life in this way sets the stage for young children to be able to recognize that just like Leo the Lion, their own Sneaky Fears put worry thoughts in their brain that make them feel nervous and scared.

In the Taming Sneaky Fears program, young children are encouraged to give their own Sneaky Fears a pet name and draw a picture of what their own Sneaky Fears look like. This represents a first step towards young children learning that their previously intimidating Sneaky Fears are not so scary after all, and that they can exert control over their Sneaky Fears. Young children learn that they can choose to ignore Sneaky Fears or talk back to Sneaky Fears and tell Sneaky Fears to leave them alone and quit bothering them (as suggested by others, e.g., Huebner, 2006). Young children learn that they can choose to Be the Boss of their Body and Be the Boss of their Brain and not let Sneaky Fears be the boss.

As with older children in traditional CBT, young children in the Sneaky Taming Fears program learn, in a step-wise manner, how to recognize their anxiety symptoms, understand when their anxiety bothers them (triggers), and manage and cope with their anxiety symptoms. In a first step, they learn how to recognize anxiety symptoms by finding out How to Be a Feeling Catcher (by doing a Body Scan to figure out what emotion they are feeling and where they are feeling the emotion in their body, and by using the Feeling Thermometer to gauge how intensely they are feeling the emotion). Second, to manage and cope with anxiety symptoms, they learn How to Be the Boss of My Body by using relaxation strategies, including Spaghetti Arms and Toes (progressive muscle relaxation), Balloon Breathing (controlled or diaphragmatic breathing), and Imagery, to make their body relax and calm down even when their body does not want to calm down. Third, young anxious children learn How to Be the Boss of My Brain (or correct cognitive distortions and replace automatic, inaccurate, and unhelpful thoughts with thoughts that are more accurate and more helpful) by (1) using the relaxation strategies to be calm enough to think clearly; then (2) visualizing the Stop sign (to make their brain so busy thinking about the shape, color, and letters of the Stop sign that their brain has no time to think about the worry or scary thoughts that Sneaky Fears try to sneak into their brain); then (3) being a Trick Catcher and catching the Tricks that Sneaky Fears play (i.e., cognitive distortions: Not Telling the Truth, Exaggerating, and Only Showing the Bad Things); and then (4) using the Trick Stoppers (or coping strategies to correct cognitive distortions: Ignore Sneaky Fears, Think Brave Thoughts, and Talk to an Adult). Fourth, young anxious children learn How to Climb Bravery Ladders (or progressive desensitization) to face and overcome their fears and show that they are becoming brave. Finally, young children learn to identify the triggers of their anxiety by recognizing situations in which their Sneaky Fears bother them the most. The ultimate goal is Taming Sneaky Fears!

6.1.1.2   Cognitive Triangle Component of Traditional CBT

Figure 6.1 illustrates the traditional cognitive triangle that shows the links among thought, feeling, and behavior. Older children, adolescents, and adults participating in traditional CBT typically learn to critically examine the automatic thought they generate when a given situation occurs and determine whether this thought is accurate (vs. inaccurate—or a cognitive distortion) and helpful (vs. unhelpful—or generating a negative feeling that negatively affects behavior). Over time, traditional CBT teaches older children, adolescents, and adults to challenge any automatic, inaccurate, and unhelpful thought and replace it with a thought that is more accurate and more helpful. This, in turn, positively affects how they feel (feeling) and what they do (behavior) in a given situation.

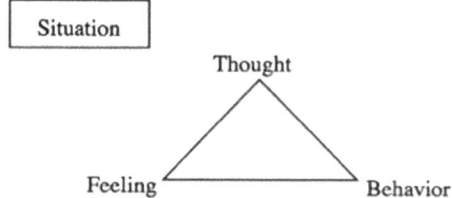

Fig. 6.1   The traditional CBT cognitive triangle

Of course, the aforementioned terminology traditionally used to explain and illustrate the interplay among thought, feeling, and behavior is quite cognitively sophisticated for four- to seven-year-old children to grasp. Nonetheless, young anxious
children can learn to recognize how their thoughts, feelings, and behaviors are inter-
related and how they can change the thought or feeling generated in a given situation
to, in turn, affect what they do (behavior). In the Taming Sneaky Fears program,
young children learn that when they feel shy, nervous, or scared (i.e., a negative
feeling) at a high level on the Feeling Thermometer (i.e., 5 or above on the 10-point
Feeling Thermometer), it usually means that their Sneaky Fears are playing their
Tricks of Not Telling the Truth, Exaggerating, and/or Only Showing the Bad Things
on their brain (i.e., putting one (or more) inaccurate and unhelpful thought(s) in their
brain). Young children learn that by being a Feeling Catcher (and doing a Body
Scan and using the Feeling Thermometer to figure out what they are feeling and how
intense the feeling is) and getting their Feeling Thermometer down to a 1 or a 2 (by
using their relaxation strategies, i.e., Spaghetti Arms and Toes, Balloon Breathing,
and Imagery), they can Be the Boss of their Body. They learn that when their Feeling
Thermometer is down to a 1 or a 2 on the 10-point Feeling Thermometer, they can
think more clearly, which makes it easier for them to use the Stop sign, be a Trick
Catcher to figure out what Trick their own Sneaky Fears are playing on their brain
(i.e., what cognitive distortion is at play), and use the Trick Stoppers (Ignore Sneaky
Fears, Think Brave Thoughts, and Talk to an Adult) to Be the Boss of their Brain (i.e.,
challenge the automatic thought or cognitive distortion). Children learn that when
they make their brain Think Brave Thoughts or Ignore Sneaky Fears (i.e., when they
generate a more accurate and helpful thought in a given situation), they feel less
shy, nervous, and scared (i.e., positively affect feeling) and, in turn, they are better
able to face and overcome the fears that they would otherwise have avoided (i.e.,
positively affect behavior). Young children also learn that when they are the Boss
of their Body and the Boss of their Brain, they can Climb their Bravery Ladder to
show that they are becoming brave, overcoming their fears, and taming their Sneaky
Fears. The parents of young anxious children also learn how the cognitive triangle
of traditional CBT and the Taming Sneaky Fears program overlap (Fig. 6.2).

THE TAMING SNEAKY FEARS PROGRAM

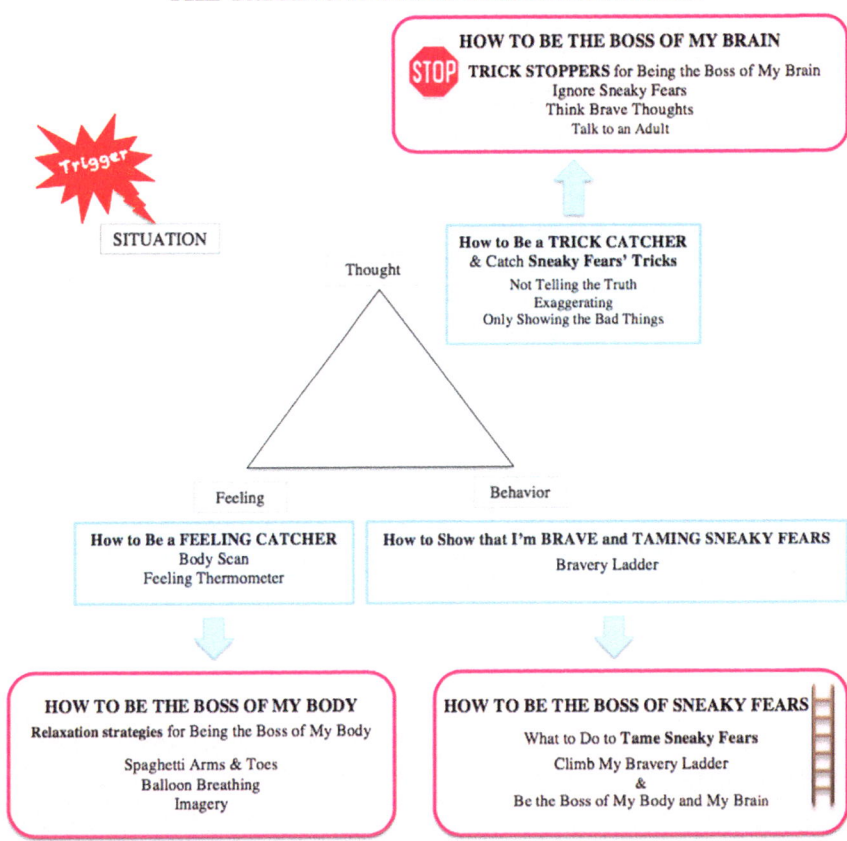

Fig. 6.2 Overlap between traditional CBT and the Taming Sneaky Fears program

6.2 Requirements for Implementation

Chapter 6 provides an overview of the Taming Sneaky Fears program along with guidelines for the implementation of the program, while Chaps. 7–11 provide step-by-step guidelines on how to implement each of the nine sessions of the Taming Sneaky Fears program in a group format, and Chap. 12 provides guidelines on how to involve school personnel as needed.[2]

---

[2]Although the Taming Sneaky Fears program was designed for use in a group format, it can also be used in individual sessions with young children and parents.

6.2.1   Who Is a Good Candidate for Participation?

Most four- to seven-year-old children who have incapacitating anxiety symptoms or a formal diagnosis of anxiety disorder are good candidates for participation in the Taming Sneaky Fears program. While most four- to seven-year-old children have fears or worries at some time or another, it is when the fears and worries become excessive and/or interfere in the day-to-day functioning of children that they become an anxiety disorder. That is, children may have an anxiety disorder when anxiety symptoms prevent them from doing age-appropriate activities such as getting to school and functioning in the school setting (e.g., speaking with a normal voice to teachers and peers, being dropped off without excessive distress), socializing with peers (e.g., going on play dates, participating in extra-curricular activities), or functioning at home (e.g., separating from parents, sleeping in their own bed). Table 1.2 (Chap. 1) lists diagnostic criteria for various anxiety disorders affecting young children while Table 6.1 describes the symptoms and primary fear or worry expressed by young anxious children. Panic disorder is not included as a diagnosis in Table 6.1 because it is virtually never diagnosed in four- to seven-year-old children, as mentioned in Chap. 1. However, young children may display panic attacks, which do not represent a psychiatric disorder per se. Panic attacks require the presence of four or more of symptoms such as, racing heartbeat, trouble catching breath, chest pain, nausea, stomachache, shaking, feeling hot and/or sweaty or cold, dizziness or lightheadedness, and tingling or numbing of fingers or other body parts.

A comprehensive and sensitively conducted clinical assessment completed with anxious young children and their parents by a qualified professional helps to identify the children's primary fear and/or worry and allows for the confirmation of an anxiety disorder diagnosis. The various assessment tools described in Chaps. 2 and 3 could be used to assist with completing a comprehensive clinical assessment. Not all children participating in the Taming Sneaky Fears program must undergo a psychiatric or psychological assessment. However, such assessments are encouraged as they help clinicians and researchers implementing the Taming Sneaky Fears program tailor the program to meet the specific needs of the participating children and ensure that the children's *primary* problem is anxiety (as opposed to a disruptive behavior disorder, autism spectrum disorder, or other disorders that are not appropriate for the Taming Sneaky Fears program). Children who do not meet all required diagnostic criteria for a DSM-5 (American Psychiatric Association, 2013) or ICD-10 (World Health Organization, 2016) anxiety disorder diagnosis but experience fears and worries that cause mild interference in their functioning or children whose symptoms of anxiety are recurrent in nature (e.g., waxing and waning nature in response to stressors) could also benefit from the Taming Sneaky Fears program (again, if their primary underlying diagnosis is not disruptive behavior disorder, autism spectrum disorder, or other disorders).

Table 6.1 Anxiety disorders—symptoms and primary fear or worry

Anxiety disorder	Symptoms[a] that interfere with functioning	Primary fear or worry
Generalized anxiety disorder	Worry excessively, more than most peers, and have trouble controlling worries Seek reassurance, but not easily reassured Somatic complaints (e.g., stomachache)	Many situations: the future, the past, friends, weather, skills and abilities, every day situations (e.g., being late, making mistakes), etc.
Social anxiety disorder	Excessive shyness, self-consciousness (e.g., think that they will do something embarrassing and people will laugh at them or make fun of them), freeze when in the spotlight Require warm-up period before can start to interact and have trouble approaching new people and new situations, raising hand in classroom to ask or answer questions, speaking on the phone, having their picture taken, using public washrooms, eating in front of people, etc. Performance anxiety	Doing or saying something silly or embarrassing in front of others or that others will laugh at them or think bad things about them
Selective mutism	Fear of being seen or heard speaking in some situations so do not speak in specific situations (e.g., school), but speak without problem in others (e.g., at home)	Voice sounds weird or funny to others
Specific phobia	Incapacitating fear or anxiety about a specific object or situation	Animal (e.g., spiders, insects, dogs) Natural environment (e.g., heights, storms, water) Blood-injection-injury (e.g., needles, invasive medical procedures)

[a]Many children with anxiety disorders have temperamental traits such as high intensity of reactions, low adaptability (e.g., trouble adapting to changes in routines and transitions), and perfectionism

Table 6.2 provides a list to assist clinicians and researchers in determining characteristics of parents and children that make them good candidates for participation in the Taming Sneaky Fears program or indicate that they should be excluded from participation.

6.2.2 Who Is Qualified to Implement the Taming Sneaky Fears Program?

The Taming Sneaky Fears program has successfully been implemented by a variety of mental health professionals, including psychiatrists, child and adolescent psychiatrists, psychologists, social workers, child and youth workers, speech and language pathologists, and trainees from these various disciplines. Parent group therapists and child group therapists may also be guidance counselors or other school mental health therapists, and other health professionals with experience working with young children, including pediatricians, family physicians, nurse practitioners, nurses, and others, as well as trainees in all these aforementioned disciplines, under supervision. To date, all therapists involved in the implementation of the Taming Sneaky Fears program have had at minimum the designation of child and youth worker, which is a three-year advanced college course focusing on the skills and knowledge required to work with children, adolescents, and families with a variety of emotional, social, behavioral, and/or mental health needs. At minimum, the equivalent training (i.e., college course focusing on working with children and youths with a variety of psycho-social-emotional needs) is required to implement the program.

Although not necessary, both parent and child group therapists benefit from having previous experience working in a group format and with young children and parents.

6.2.3 Where Can the Taming Sneaky Fears Program Be Implemented?

The Taming Sneaky Fears group CBT program has successfully been implemented in tertiary psychiatric settings and community mental health agencies. The program could be implemented in a variety of clinical settings such as psychiatric, psychological, and other health and mental health settings. Additionally, the program may be implemented in school settings by school social workers, psychologists, or counselors with experience in children's mental health.

To date, the Taming Sneaky Fears program has been implemented mostly as a group treatment program in clinical and research settings. However, as previously mentioned, clinicians have successfully used the program in individual sessions with

Table 6.2 Characteristics of parents and children who are good candidates for participation in the Taming Sneaky Fears program or who should be excluded from participation

	Good candidates	Exclusionary characteristics[a]
Parents	Understand and speak fluently the language in which the program is offered	Lack of fluency in the language in which the program is offered and/or difficulties with literacy
	Are the children's primary caregivers	Custody and access dispute
	Willing to discuss self and child in a group format	Unresolved child protection matter
	Available for program – One parent must attend all sessions – Live in close enough proximity to commit to regular attendance	Unable to commit to attending all sessions
	Willing to engage in the treatment program and implement recommended strategies at home	Too anxious to function in a group setting
	Amenable to change	Acute or poorly managed mental health or addiction problem (e.g., depression, psychosis, posttraumatic stress disorder, substance abuse)
Children	Between ages of four and seven years	Eight years or older; younger than four[b]
	Have a primary anxiety disorder or symptoms of anxiety that cause at least mild interference with functioning and/or are recurrent in nature	Primary diagnosis is autism spectrum disorder, posttraumatic stress disorder, or a non-anxiety disorder
	Of average intelligence (based on clinical impression, not formal testing)	Brain injury or significant developmental delay
	Understand and speak fluently the language in which the program is offered	Too aggressive
	Able to attend and focus sufficiently	Too disruptive
	May have co-morbid diagnoses of attention deficit hyperactivity disorder or oppositional defiant disorder, but the primary problem is anxiety	Do not have a primary caregiver

[a]Parents and/or children should not receive other concurrent mental health counseling, but other types of interventions can co-occur, such as, for the children, Occupational Therapy, Physiotherapy, Speech and Language Therapy, participation in psychological assessments, psychiatric assessment or follow up, and for the parents, psychiatric assessment or follow up, addiction support programs such as Alcoholic Anonymous, Narcotic Anonymous, etc.

[b]To date, the Taming Sneaky Fears program has been implemented mostly with four- to seven-year-old children. However, clinicians have successfully used aspects of the program in individual sessions with children as young as three years old, in conjunction with separate sessions with their parents. Therefore, clinicians and researchers could consider using aspects of the Taming Sneaky Fears program with some (carefully selected) children as young as three years old

young anxious children, in conjunction with separate sessions with their parents. Therefore, clinicians and researchers could consider using the program as individual sessions with young children and having additional sessions with their parents to provide parents with the necessary information about the parent program.

6.2.4 When to Implement the Taming Sneaky Fears Program?

Given the young age of the children, consideration should be given to running the Taming Sneaky Fears program during the morning or early to mid-afternoon as young four- to seven-year-old children generally absorb information better early during the day rather than in the late afternoon or early evening.

6.3 Program Overview

6.3.1 Duration and Frequency

The Taming Sneaky Fears program consists of nine 45- to 50-minute sessions: one Introduction Session (for parents only) followed by eight parent group and child group sessions that are held concurrently in separate rooms. Typically, the sessions are held once weekly. However, the sessions could be held more frequently (e.g., twice per week) as needed, for example, to accommodate delivery of the program as a summer program.

6.3.2 Therapists-to-Parents and Therapists-to-Children Ratio

It is feasible to run the parent group with only one parent group therapist. However, it is ideal for two parent group therapists to be available to ensure adequate coverage throughout the program (i.e., should the lead parent group therapist be ill or otherwise unable to attend, a second parent group therapist is available to take over). Ideally, a minimum of four and a maximum of 18 parents participate in the parent group. Although both parents (in a two-parent family) may attend the parent group, oftentimes only one parent can commit to assiduous attendance. Ideally, at least one parent attends all sessions in order to ensure that at least one parent receives the full curriculum. Clinical experience suggests that families with parents who alternate attendance at the parent group may not benefit from the program as much as families with at least one parent attending all sessions (with the other parent also attending all sessions, or dropping in whenever possible, or not attending at all). In addition, sporadic attendance by parents can be disruptive to the other group participants. Therefore, two-parent families are encouraged to designate one parent to attend all sessions and have the other parent attend whenever possible.

Ideally, the child group consists of six to nine children with two to three child group therapists. It is difficult to run a group with fewer than four children attending and difficult to accommodate more than nine children. Given the young age of the children participating in the Taming Sneaky Fears program and the relatively high prevalence of separation anxiety in this young age group, the child group requires two child group therapists at a minimum and depending upon the number of children attending the group and their anxiety diagnoses, more child group therapists might be needed.

6.3.3 Setting and Materials

The Taming Sneaky Fears program is implemented in two separate, large enough rooms to comfortably accommodate all participants and therapists. Ideally, these two rooms are located in close proximity of one another.

6.3.3.1 Parent Group Room

The parent group room contains a table (or other surface for parents to take notes) and comfortable chairs set up around the table. On the table, the following items are available at each session: (1) name tags for parents and therapists to re-use at each session (ideally, each name tag has the parent's name printed in large font at the top and the child's name printed underneath the parent's names in smaller font, but large enough to be read from a distance); (2) extra copies of the Parent Manual[3] for parents who forget to bring their Parent Manual; (3) extra pens (for parents to use as needed); (4) copies of the various recommended books and DVDs (listed in Sect. 7.3); and (5) a box of tissues.

In addition, the following items (summarized in Table 6.3) are available in the parent group room at each session: (1) white board and/or flip chart and markers (if a white board is used, information needs to be recorded in some fashion to use at future sessions); (2) dry erase markers, dry erase solvent, and sponge wipe for laminated materials ; (3) large laminated picture of a blank Bravery Ladder that

---

[3]The Parent Manual is provided as one of the Supplementary Materials with this chapter.

can be written on, erased, and re-used and is the approximate size of a white board or flip chart (Fig. 28 in the Parent Manual); and (4) laminated copies (on regular 8″ by 11″ size paper) of the illustration showing the overlap between traditional CBT and the Taming Sneaky Fears program (Fig. 6.2 of this chapter or Fig. 3 of the Parent Manual), the What to Do to Help list (Fig. 4 of the Parent Manual), and the Feeling Thermometer (Fig. 8 of the Parent Manual). Table 6.3 summarizes the various aforementioned materials and details about setting that are recommended in the implementation of the Taming Sneaky Fears group CBT program with parents.

6.3.3.2 Child Group Room

Ideally, the child group room is large enough to accommodate all participants. Comfortable chairs for all children and child group therapists are positioned in a small circle. Alternatively, the children and child group therapists can sit on the floor on a suitable mat. Two small tables (or other surfaces) are available, one to set up the snack and one for the children to use when they complete their craft at each session. Pre-printed, stick-on name tags for children and child group therapists are available. Additional materials required at each child session include: (1) *Taming Sneaky Fears—Leo the Lion's story of bravery & Inside Leo's den: The workbook* (Benoit & Monga, 2018a, b; one per child) in order for each child to complete the various drawings that are part of the workbook section of the book during Craft Time; (2) the Supplementary Child Workbook[4] that contains the additional crafts to complete during Craft Time at some of the child sessions; the child group therapists bring both of these workbooks to each session for the children to use as needed and these workbooks are given to the children to take home at the final graduation session; (3) crayons and markers in a basket or other container; (4) stickers (to use for incentives or rewards); (5) white board and/or flip chart and markers (if a white board is used, information needs to be recorded in some fashion to use at future sessions); (6) dry erase markers, dry erase solvent, and sponge wipe for laminated materials; (7) large, full body, animal puppets, including puppets to portray the five main story characters: Leo the Lion,[5] Ellie the Elephant,[6] Sneaky Fears,[7] Missy Mistake,[8] and Ms. Priya the Panther,[9] and four to six additional animal puppets[10] (the number of additional puppets depends upon the number of children in the group as each child uses a puppet at each session; the puppets for Leo

---

[4]The Supplementary Child Workbook is provided as one of the Supplementary Materials with this chapter.

[5]Leo the Lion: Folkmanis full body lion puppet number 2889.

[6]Ellie the Elephant: Folkmanis full body elephant puppet number 2534.

[7]Sneaky Fears: *Two* Folkmanis full body gray fox puppets number 3032.

[8]Missy Mistake: Folkmanis Fire Dragon puppet number 3054.

[9]Ms. Priya the Panther: Folkmanis Black Cat puppet number 2987.

[10]Any of the following Folkmanis full body puppets could be used for the four to six additional puppets (puppet number in brackets): Chimpanzee (2877), snowy owl (2236), ostrich (3026), tiger (2869) baboon (2914), peacock (2539), small panda bear (2364), koala (3057), sloth (2927),

Table 6.3 Setting and materials

	Parent group	Child group
Large room to comfortably accommodate all participants	✔	✔
Comfortable chairs for participants (positioned in a small circle in the child group; around the table in the parent group)	✔	✔
White board and/or flip chart and markers (if white board is used, information is recorded in some fashion to use at future sessions)	✔	✔
Dry erase markers, dry erase solvent, and sponge wipe for laminated materials (if a white board is used)	✔	✔
Name tags with pre-printed names—stick-on for children for each session; pin-on for parents to re-use at each session (parent name in large font at the top and child name in smaller font but large enough to be read from a distance at the bottom)	✔	✔
Snack list[a] (if parents are providing snack for the children)	✔	
Table so participants can comfortably take notes	✔	
Parent Manual (one for each parent distributed at the Introduction Session, plus extra copies at each subsequent session for parents who forget to bring their Parent Manual; provided as one of the Supplementary Materials with this chapter)	✔	
Pens for parents to use as needed	✔	
Laminated copy (on regular 8″ × 11″ size paper) of: 1. The Taming Sneaky Fears program (Fig. 6.2 of this chapter or Fig. 3 of the Parent Manual)	✔	
2. What to Do to Help list (Fig. 4 of the Parent Manual)	✔	
3. Feeling Thermometer (Fig. 8 of the Parent Manual)	✔	
Children's story & companion workbook: *Taming Sneaky Fears—Leo the Lion's story of bravery & Inside Leo's den: The workbook* (Benoit & Monga, 2018a, b)		✔
Supplementary Child Workbook—one per child (provided as one of the Supplementary Materials with this chapter)		✔
Animal puppets, including the five main story characters: Leo the Lion, Ellie the Elephant, Sneaky Fears, Missy Mistake, and Ms. Priya the Panther, and as many puppets as there are children in the group; all puppets except Sneaky Fears and Missy Mistake (that are for the exclusive use of the child group therapists at specific child sessions) are easily accessible, but partially hidden at the beginning of each session so children do not gravitate towards them when they enter the group room		✔
Stickers (or other form of incentive/reward) at each session to be used for incentive/reward for practicing strategies between sessions or participating in session		✔

(continued)

Table 6.3 (continued)

	Parent group	Child group
Large (size of a flip chart) laminated materials that can be written on, erased, and re-used 1. Bravery Ladder (Fig. 28 of the Parent Manual) 2. Body outline (for Body Scan; Fig. 6 of the Parent Manual) 3. Feeling Thermometer (Fig. 8 of the Parent Manual)	✔	✔ ✔ ✔
Laminated pictures/drawings of each step of My First Bravery Ladder for Being Friendly with __(a specific person) (modified Fig. 25 of the Parent Manual) with Velcro - large enough to be placed on each step of a large Bravery Ladder (see Sections "Groups of Children Who Have Various Fears" and "Groups of Children with Selective Mutism and/or Social Anxiety Disorder" for details)[b]		✔
Small table or other surface for children to do craft		✔
Crayons and markers at each session		✔
Snack[c]—be mindful of food intolerance or allergies		✔
Small toy or stuffed animals for children to use when learning Balloon Breathing		✔
Story book or game (e.g., a Franklin the Turtle Story or Matching Pairs game) for use during Snack Time, if time permits		✔
Graduation certificate (Fig. 11.1)		✔

[a]If the parents are providing the snack for the children, a snack list is generated with the parents at the Introduction Session (to determine which parents bring the snack at which session) and at each subsequent parent session, the parent group therapists remind the parents of who is bringing snack to the next session
[b]For use with children during C-Sessions 6 and 7 (Fig. 25 from the Parent Manual is modified as described in Sections "Groups of Children Who Have Various Fears" and "Groups of Children with Selective Mutism and/or Social Anxiety Disorder")
[c]If the therapists are providing the snack at each child session, an appropriate snack (e.g. granola bar and juice box) is available for each child at each child session

the Lion, Ellie the Elephant, and Ms. Priya the Panther can be used by the children during sessions; however, the Sneaky Fears and Missy Mistake puppets are used by the child group therapists only during the Story Time portions of specific child sessions); (8) a story book (other than the children's story section of the Benoit and Monga's *Taming Sneaky Fears—Leo's the Lion's story of bravery & Inside Leo's den: The workbook*) or game typically enjoyed by four- to seven-year-old children to be used at the end of each session to encourage socialization if time permits (e.g., a Franklin the Turtle Story or Matching Pairs game); and (9) snack such as fruit or granola bar and drink provided by therapists or parents (see Sect. 6.3.3.3).

chameleon (2215), bob cat (2199), ant eater (2973), lion mountain (3045), slow loris (3072), armadillo (3043), camel (2979), parrot (2592), macaw (3078).

In addition, various materials are needed at specific sessions in the child group, including (1) a large blank body outline (e.g., Fig. 6 of the Parent Manual), approximately the size of a white board or flip chart (or a large body outline can be drawn on the flip chart) for use in child sessions (C-Sessions) 1 and 2; (2) small toys or stuffed animals for the children to use when learning Balloon Breathing at C-Session 2 and each subsequent session; (3) the Sneaky Fears puppets starting in C-Session 2 and the Missy Mistake puppet starting in C-Session 6; (4) a blank laminated Feeling Thermometer (Fig. 8 of the Parent Manual) the size of a white board or flip chart (or a Feeling Thermometer can be drawn on the flip chart at C-Session 5 and each subsequent session; (6) a large laminated Bravery Ladder (Fig. 28 of the Parent Manual) along with laminated stick-on illustrations of the 'steps to being friendly' with Velcro on the back of each illustration (as detailed in Sect. 10.3.3.1.1); and (7) a graduation certificate for each child at C-Session 8 (e.g., Fig. 11.1). Table 6.3 summarizes the various aforementioned details about setting and materials that are recommended in the implementation of the Taming Sneaky Fears group CBT program with children.

6.3.3.3 Snack

Snack could be provided either by the professionals running the group or by the parents attending the group program. If parents provide the snack, a list of which parent is responsible for bringing the snack at which session is established during the Introduction Session (Sect. 7.2.4). Prior to the end of each parent session, the parent group therapists remind the parents of who is responsible for bringing the snack to the following session. Socioeconomic and other variables can help to determine whether snack is provided by the professionals running the program or by parents attending the group. Snack typically consists of healthy and nutritious foods such as cheese and crackers, cut-up fruit, or a granola bar along with a juice box or water. Allergies, other food tolerances, and/or specific dietary requirements must be taken into consideration when determining the snack. The role of Snack Time is detailed in Sect. 8.4.6.1.

6.3.4 Contents

As seen in Fig. 6.3, children and parents participating in the Taming Sneaky Fears program learn three main concepts and related skills over the eight group sessions following the Introduction Session, i.e., How to Be the Boss of My Body, How to Be the Boss of My Brain, and How to Climb Bravery Ladders. Children (and their parents) discover How to Be the Boss of My Body by learning two skills: (1) How to Be a Feeling Catcher by doing a Body Scan and using the Feeling Thermometer and (2) how to use relaxation strategies, including Spaghetti Arms and Toes, Balloon Breathing, and Imagery. With the parents, the concept of How to Be the Boss of My Body and related skills are covered during parent session (P-Session) 1 and

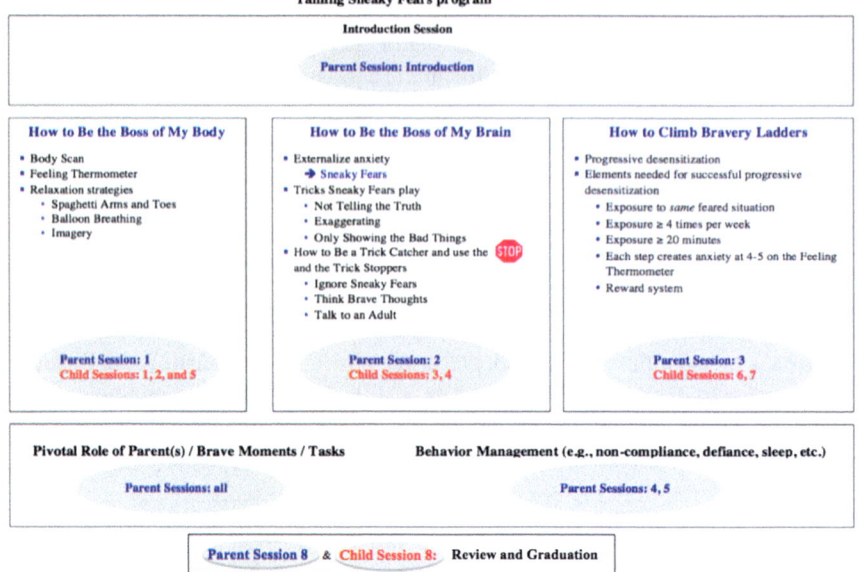

Fig. 6.3 Overview of concepts and skills covered in the Taming Sneaky Fears program

frequently revisited during subsequent sessions. With the children, the concept and related skills are covered over multiple sessions because young children require practice and repetition to master how to do a Body Scan (child sessions (C-Sessions) 1, 2, and subsequent sessions), how to use the Feeling Thermometer (C-Session 5 and subsequent sessions), and how to correctly use the relaxation strategies (C-Session 1 and every subsequent session).

Table 6.4 provides a detailed outline of the topics covered during the Introduction Session and each of the subsequent eight sessions of the Taming Sneaky Fears program, including the suggested number of minutes devoted to each topic or activity in the parent and child groups.

As seen in Table 6.4, the Introduction Session differs from all subsequent sessions. Chapter 7 focuses on this Introduction Session and provides step-by-step guidelines to implement it successfully. Chapters 8–11 focus on subsequent sessions.

Table 6.4 The Taming Sneaky Fears group CBT program at a glance—Format and outline of topics covered at each session

Session[a]	Parent group[b]		Child group[b]	
	Minutes		Minutes	
Introduction	10–15	Welcome, introductions, and overview of the child component of program (all parents and therapists are present; led by one child group therapist, then the child group therapists leave)		
	30–35	Overview of the parent and child programs (led by parent group therapists after the child group therapists depart) Psychoeducation • Anxiety Disorders • Overlap between CBT and the Taming Sneaky Fears program • What to Do to Help Brave moments and effective praise		
1	5	Introduction of children	5	Introduction of children
	5	Debrief around separation	10	Circle Time and Story Time—Story[c] Chapter 1—Meet Leo the Lion and discussion of story
	10	Brave moments and effective praise	5	Purpose, rules, and name of the group
	30	How to Be a Feeling Catcher • Body Scan • Feeling Thermometer How to Be the Boss of My Body • Spaghetti Arms and Toes • Balloon Breathing • Imagery	15	How to Be a Feeling Catcher • Body Scans for happy and mad/angry How to Be the Boss of My Body • Spaghetti Arms and Toes
			10	Craft Time
			5	Snack Time
	<1	Wrap up—when child group therapist enters the parent group room, parent group session ends	<1	Wrap up—one child therapist goes to parent room to signal end of session

(continued)

Table 6.4 (continued)

Session[a]	Parent group[b]		Child group[b]	
	Minutes		Minutes	
2	5	Parents volunteer examples of brave moments and effective praise	5	Circle Time—reintroduction of children, review of events that might have happened to the children since the previous session, and review of topics covered in the previous session
	5	Review of other tasks	10	Story Time—Story[c] Chapter 2 and discussion of story

	30–40	How to Be a Trick Catcher and catch the Tricks Sneaky Fears play
		• Not Telling the Truth
		• Exaggerating
		• Only Showing the Bad Things
		How to Be the Boss of My Brain
		• Use the Stop sign
		• Use the Trick Stoppers:
		  – Ignore Sneaky Fears
		  – Think Brave Thoughts
		  – Talk to an Adult
			15	How to Be the Boss of My Body
				• Balloon Breathing
				• Imagery
				How to Be a Feeling Catcher
				• Body Scans for nervous/scared and shy

			10	Craft Time
			5	Snack Time
	<1	Wrap up	<1	Wrap up
3	5–10	Parents volunteer examples of brave moments and effective praise	5–10	Circle Time—review of events that might have happened to the children since the previous session, topics covered at the previous session, and relaxation strategies
	5–10	Review of other tasks	10	Story Time—Story[c] Chapter 3—Meet Sneaky Fears and discussion of story

	30–40	How to Climb Bravery Ladders (to overcome fears)
		How to manage excessive worries
			15	How to Be a Trick Catcher
				• Trick #1: Not Telling the Truth
				How to Be the Boss of My Brain:
				• Use the Stop sign
				• Use the Trick Stoppers
				  – Ignore Sneaky Fears
				  – Think Brave Thoughts

			10	Craft Time
			5	Snack Time
	<1	Wrap up	<1	Wrap up

(continued)

Table 6.4 (continued)

Session[a]	Parent group[b]		Child group[b]	
	Minutes		Minutes	
4	5	How to manage behavior	5–10	Circle Time—review of events that might have happened to the children since the previous session, topics covered at the previous session, and relaxation strategies
	45	Watch the *1-2-3 Magic* DVD	10	Story Time—Story[c] Chapter 4 and discussion of story
			15	How to be a Trick Catcher • Trick #2: Exaggerating • Trick #3: Only Showing the Bad Things How to Be the Boss of My Brain: • Use the Trick Stopper – Talk to an Adult
			10	Craft Time
			5	Snack Time
	<1	Wrap up	<1	Wrap up
	*Child group therapists meet with each child's parent(s) for five minutes **at the end of Session 4** and (as needed) **immediately prior to the beginning of Session 5** to provide and receive feedback on each child's progress*			
5	*Child group therapists meet with each child's parent(s) for five minutes **at the end of Session 4** and (as needed) **immediately prior to the beginning of Session 5** to provide and receive feedback on each child's progress*			
	5–10	Parents volunteer examples of brave moments and effective praise	5–10	Circle Time—review of events that might have happened to the children since the previous session, topics covered in the previous session, and relaxation strategies
	5–10	Review of other tasks	10	Story Time—Story[c] Chapter 5 and discussion of story
	30–40	Common problem: Sleep Importance of humor Bravery Ladders—Review	15	How to Be a Feeling Catcher • Feeling Thermometer
			10	Craft Time
			5	Snack Time
	<1	Wrap up	<1	Wrap up

(continued)

Table 6.4 (continued)

Session[a]	Parent group[b]		Child group[b]	
	Minutes		Minutes	
6	5–10	Parents volunteer examples of brave moments and effective praise	5–10	Circle Time—review of events that might have happened to the children since the previous session, topics covered at the previous sessions, and relaxation strategies
	5–10	Review of other tasks	10	Story Time—Story[c] Chapter 6 and discussion of story
	30–40	Review of materials covered to date	15	How to Climb Bravery Ladders
			10	Craft Time
			5	Snack Time
	<1	Wrap up	<1	Wrap up
7	5–10	Parents volunteer for brave moments and effective praise	5–10	Circle Time—review of events that might have happened to the children since the previous session, topics covered at the previous sessions, and relaxation strategies
	5–10	Review other homework	10	Story Time—Story[c] Chapter 7 and discussion of story
	30–40	Review session	15	How to Climb Bravery Ladders
			10	Craft Time
			5	Snack Time
	<1	Wrap up	<1	Wrap up
8[d]	20	Review session	5	Circle Time—review of events that might have happened to the children since the previous session, topics covered at the previous sessions, and relaxation strategies
			10	Story Time—story[c] Chapter 8 and discussion of story
			10	Review of all concepts
	15	Children come in for graduation	15	Children go to parent group room for graduation

[a]45- to 50-minutes sessions: children and parent groups run concurrently, but in separate rooms
[b]Ideally, the parent and child group rooms are in close proximity
[c]Children's story section of *Taming Sneaky Fears—Leo the Lion's story of bravery & Inside Leo's den: The workbook* (Benoit & Monga, 2018a, b)
[d]Session 8 lasts 40 minutes with the children coming to the parents' room after 25 minutes for graduation
<:less than

References

American Psychiatric Association. (2013). *Diagnostic and statistical manual of mental disorders* (5th ed.). Washington, DC: American Psychiatric Association.

Benoit, D., & Monga, S. (2018a). *Apprivoiser les Peurs-pas-fines—L'histoire de bravoure de Léo le lionceau & Dans la tanière de Léo: Le cahier de travail*. Victoria, British Columbia: FriesenPress.

Benoit, D., & Monga, S. (2018b). *Taming Sneaky Fears—Leo the Lion's story of bravery & inside Leo's den: The workbook*. Victoria, British Columbia: FriesenPress.

Huebner, D. (2006). *What to do when you worry too much—A kid's guide to overcoming anxiety*. Washington, DC: Magination Press.

World Health Organization (2016). *The ICD-10 classification of mental and behavioural disorders: Clinical descriptions and diagnostic guidelines*. Geneva: World Health Organization.

Chapter 7
The Taming Sneaky Fears Program: Introduction Session

7.1 Purpose of the Introduction Session

The purpose of the Introduction Session is threefold. First, it introduces parents to the child and parent group therapists and vice versa. Second, it allows the child group therapists to provide a brief, 10- to 15-minute description of some aspects of the child group component of the Taming Sneaky Fears program to the parents, prepare them for Session 1 with the children, and identify and problem solve anticipated difficulties with the separation between parents and children that takes place in Session 1. Third, it allows the parent group therapists to distribute the Parent Manual,[1] provide an overview of the parent group component of the program, discuss rules and expectations of group participation, deliver psychoeducation (anxiety and anxiety disorders, overlap between CBT and the Taming Sneaky Fears program), discuss the various materials used and recommended for the program (summarized in Sect. 7.2.4), and address questions or concerns parents might have.

7.2 Step-by-Step Guidelines to Implement the Introduction Session

7.2.1 Days or Weeks Prior to the Introduction Session

Several days or weeks prior to the Introduction Session, the lead parent and child group therapists ensure that (1) parents are contacted to confirm the start date, time, and location of the Introduction Session and know to come without their children;

---

[1] The Parent Manual is available as one of the Supplementary Materials in Chap 6.

© Springer Nature Switzerland AG 2018
S. Monga and D. Benoit, *Assessing and Treating Anxiety Disorders in Young Children*, https://doi.org/10.1007/978-3-030-04939-3_7

(2) assessment information on the children (documenting their anxiety diagnoses and clinical symptoms) is available; and (3) all rooms and materials needed for the Introduction Session are available. From the materials listed in Table 6.3, the parent group therapists need enough copies of the Parent Manual to distribute to each parent, pens for parents to use as needed, one laminated copy of Fig. 6.2 (or Fig. 3 in the Parent Manual that illustrates the overlap between traditional CBT and the Taming Sneaky Fears program), and one laminated copy of Fig. 4 in the Parent Manual (the What to Do to Help list).

Prior to the Introduction Session, the parent group therapists determine who covers what materials during the session and familiarize themselves with the materials to be covered ahead of time, so as to not read verbatim from the Parent Manual, although they might find it helpful to point at, and even read, brief sections verbatim. Most of the information the parent group therapists need to prepare for the Introduction (and all subsequent sessions) is included in the Parent Manual. In preparing for the group sessions, the parent group therapists might wish to familiarize themselves with the various reference materials recommended to parents (last page of the Parent Manual).

7.2.2 On the Day of the Introduction Session

On the day of the Introduction Session, all parent and child group therapists meet for approximately 20 minutes before the Introduction Session begins to set up the parent group room with all the needed materials (summarized in Table 6.3), review information about participants (e.g., parents' and children's names, children's ages, anxiety diagnoses or anxiety symptoms, and associated symptoms such as sleep problems, oppositional and defiant behavior, separation difficulties), and clarify each of the parent and child group therapists' roles in the upcoming Introduction Session. Table 7.1 is an excerpt from Table 6.4 and summarizes the format and outline of topics covered during the Introduction Session.

7.2.3 Introduction Session—Part A (Child Group Therapist Led)

At the predetermined start time for the Introduction Session, at least one of the parent and/or child group therapists greets the parents in the waiting area and brings them to the parent group room. When all parents and all child and parent group therapists are in the parent group room, one of the child group therapists takes the lead and completes the following tasks:

1. Asks the parents, if this has not already taken place, to find their name tag on the table and put it on (all child and parent group therapists already have their name tags on).

Table 7.1 Format and outline of topics covered during the Introduction Session (excerpt from Table 6.4)

Session[a]	Parent group	
	Minutes	
Introduction	10–15	Welcome, introductions, and overview of the child component of program (all parents and therapists are present; led by one child group therapist, then the child group therapists leave)
	30–35	Overview of the parent and child programs (led by parent group therapists after the child group therapists depart) Psychoeducation • Anxiety disorders • Overlap between CBT and the Taming Sneaky Fears program • What to Do to Help Brave moments and effective praise

[a]session is 45-50 minutes.

2. Welcomes the parents.
3. Introduces self and the child and parent group therapists (alternatively, the therapists could introduce themselves).
4. Invites the parents to introduce themselves by saying their name and their child's name and age.
5. Informs the parents that the child group therapists will spend ten to 15 minutes with them before leaving and letting the parent group therapists take over.
6. Asks the parents if they have told their children about the group, and if they have, invites them to share what they have told their children. Parents are informed that it is best for the children to know that they are coming to some type of extracurricular program where they will be with other children, hear stories, do crafts, and eat a snack. However, the timing of when to tell the children about the group is up to the parents as parents know best if their children benefit from knowing a week in advance or are best told the night before or the morning of the event.
7. Answers the parents' questions pertaining to what to tell their children about the group.
8. Describes Session 1, the first session with the children, explaining that:

   • After all parents, children, and therapists come into the child group room, a child group therapist will welcome everyone and introduce all the therapists, then read out loud one child name at a time from the stick-on name tags, approach that child while asking permission to place the name tag on the child's shirt and asking the child's age and grade in school.
   • After all the children are introduced, one of the child group therapists will call out, "It's story time," which is the signal for all of the parents to smile,

look calm, and promptly follow the parent group therapists out of the child group room to the parent group room.

9. Asks the parents if they anticipate their children will have difficulties with the separation (this information is useful for the therapists so they can be ready to take on a more active role at Session 1 with dyads that might struggle with the separation, as needed).
10. Explains that the child group therapists are experienced and can manage children who may have difficulties with the separation.
11. Explains to parents that it is easier for children to know that there will be a separation early in Session 1 and that when children are aware that a separation will take place, they are generally less distressed at the separation.
12. Informs the parents that after today's session, they will see one or more child group therapists again:

    - At the beginning of each session as at least one child group therapist greets them and their children in the waiting area and directs them to their respective room.
    - At the end of each group session when a child group therapist comes to the parent group room to give a ten-second summary of the session, which is the signal for the parents and parent therapists to end the session promptly ("Today, we talked about ____. The children are ready for you to pick them up").
    - At the end of each session as parents come to get their children in the child group room.
    - Halfway through the program when one of the child group therapists meets each of the children's parent(s) to provide brief feedback on how their child is doing in the child group; this is also an opportunity for parents to let the child group therapist (and thus all therapists) know about any changes noted in their children at home and school since the start of the group program. Generally, the child group therapists take approximately five minutes with each set of parents immediately after Session 4 is completed or before Session 5 begins to provide this feedback.
    - At the very last session, for the graduation ceremony.

13. Answers questions the parents may have and then informs them that the child group therapists are leaving and the parent group therapists are taking over for the rest of this Introduction Session.

7.2.4   Introduction Session—Part B (Parent Group Therapist Led)

When the child group therapists leave, the lead parent group therapist takes the lead and completes the following tasks:

1. Distributes the Parent Manuals (one Parent Manual per parent).
2. Instructs the parents to follow along as all the information that is discussed during the Introduction Session is included in the Parent Manual.
3. Provides an orientation to the Parent Manual by:

   - Pointing out the Table of Contents and mentioning that it provides a brief overview of what topics are covered during each session of the Taming Sneaky Fears group program.
   - Directing the parents' attention to the last page of the Parent Manual, which provides a list of recommended resources for parents (ideally, a copy of these various resources are available and parents are encouraged to look through the materials during the Introduction Session, if they wish).
   - Indicating that all the materials discussed at each session, including today's session, are included in the Parent Manual.
   - Mentioning that we are not going to read verbatim every word that is written in the Parent Manual during each group session; we encourage parents to read on their own, in between sessions, all the materials in preparation for each session and for review after each session.

4. Asks the parents to turn to page 1 of the Parent Manual and provides an 'Overview of the Child Group Sessions' by:

   - Mentioning that the goals and objectives of the child group sessions are listed on page 1 and refer to concepts and skills that they, as parents, and their children will learn as part of the Taming Sneaky Fears program.
   - Holding the laminated (page-size) copy of Fig. 3 of the Parent Manual (The Taming Sneaky Fears program[2]), while pointing out to the parent the page number where parents can find Fig. 3 in the Parent Manual.
   - Explaining briefly (two or three minutes) that:
     - The Taming Sneaky Fears program is based on Cognitive Behavior Therapy (CBT), which the gray inside triangle of Fig. 3 linking thought, feeling and behavior illustrates.
     - The concepts and terminology used in traditional CBT are complex and abstract and not easily understood by four- to seven-year-old children.
     - The sections in blue and pink of Fig. 3 relate to the list of Goals and Objectives listed on page 1 of the Parent Manual and describe the terminology used in the Taming Sneaky Fears program to make abstract and complex CBT concepts and skills easier for four- to seven-year-old children to understand and learn (here, the parent group therapist mentions that parents and children will learn How to Be a Feeling Catcher by using a Body Scan and the Feeling Thermometer; How to Be the Boss of My Body by using the relaxation strategies, Spaghetti Arms and Toes, Balloon Breathing, and Imagery; How to Be a Trick Catcher and Catch the three Tricks (or cognitive distortions) that Sneaky Fears play, Not Telling the

---

[2]This is also Fig. 6.2 of this book.

Truth, Exaggerating, and Only Showing the Bad Things; How to Be the Boss of My Brain by using the Stop sign and the Trick Stoppers, Ignore Sneaky Fears, Think Brave Thoughts, and Talk to an Adult; and How to Climb Bravery Ladders to overcome fears. The program also promotes social skills.

5. Provides an overview of the format of each child session (and points out the page number where this information is found in the Parent Manual), by mentioning only that each group session is divided into four parts: each session starts with Circle Time, followed by Story Time, Craft Time, and Snack Time.

6. Reviews briefly (one minute) what the child group therapist said about Session 1 with the children (and points out the page number where this information is found in the Parent Manual), emphasizing that:

   - When parents hear one of the child group therapists say, "It's story time" (which should occur within five or so minutes of the start of Session 1), it is their cue to smile, look calm and in control, regardless of the child's reaction, and follow the parent group therapist(s) out of the room quickly.
   - The child group therapists are experienced and take an active role in helping children separate from their parents as needed.

7. Points at Table 1 (and indicates the page number where Table 1 is located in the Parent Manual), invites parents to read Table 1 in more detail, on their own, after the session, and briefly mentions that Table 1:

   - Provides a detailed outline of topics covered in each parent session and each child session.
   - Shows that parents learn the various concepts and skills one or more sessions before the children do; because of this, we ask that parents refrain from bringing up specific concepts and terminology with the children until these are covered during the child group sessions; we will begin each parent group session by mentioning what the children are learning in their own child group sessions.

8. Asks parents to turn to the section pertaining to the 'Overview of the Parent Group Sessions' (indicating the page number where this section is located in the Parent Manual) and proceeds by going over each of the 16 items listed under 'General Information and Rules' (adding, removing, or modifying items to meet the needs of specific parent groups or settings, as needed); a special emphasis is placed on identifying all children with food intolerances, food allergies, and/or specific dietary requirements[3] (the parent group therapists transmit this infor-

---

[3]If parents provide the snack for Snack Time at each child session, the parent group therapists generate a list of which parents are responsible for bringing the snack at which session during the Introduction Session and remind parents of who is responsible for bringing the snack at each subsequent session. In addition, examples of an appropriate snack are discussed with parents. Additional details can be found in Sect. 6.3.3.3.

mation to the child group therapists at the end of the Introduction Session when all parent group and child group therapists meet for a few minutes to debrief).

9. Directs the parents' attention to the next section of the Parent Manual pertaining to 'Psychoeducation' (indicating the page number where this section is located in the Parent Manual) and proceeds by indicating:

- The difference between normative anxiety and an anxiety disorder, i.e., all humans feel anxious at some point; anxiety becomes an anxiety *disorder* when it interferes with a person's functioning at home, school (or work), and in social situations.
- That the Parent Manual contains a list and brief description of the five most common anxiety disorders seen in four- to seven-year old children (separation anxiety disorder, specific phobia, generalized anxiety disorder, social anxiety disorder, and selective mutism); the parent group therapist who is in charge of covering this section invites the parents to read the information on the various anxiety disorders on their own, after the group.

10. Directs the parents' attention to the next section of the Parent Manual pertaining to 'Factors Contributing to Anxiety' (indicating the page number where this section is located in the Parent Manual) and proceeds by using Fig. 1 (and asking parents to focus on Fig. 1) to describe that:

- Two main factors are usually (not always) prerequisites for the development of an anxiety disorder:
  - *Genetic factors* (as there is often a positive family history for anxiety disorders in families of children with anxiety disorders).
  - *Temperamental traits* (such as high intensity of reactions—as in 'drama queens,' low adaptability—with children resisting changes in routines, perfectionism, sensory sensitivities).
- Many children might have genetic factors and temperamental traits that place them at risk for an anxiety disorder, but will not develop an anxiety disorder, in part because
  - *Stress* is often needed to trigger an anxiety disorder (stress for a young child can be obvious—such as the birth of a sibling or parental separation—or quite subtle—such as a change in season).
  - The *quality of the caregiver-child relationship* protects a child from developing an anxiety disorder (and here the parent group therapist provides a summary of the description of secure attachment between child and caregiver as provided in the Parent Manual).

11. Directs the parents' attention to the next section of the Parent Manual, 'Typical Responses to Anxiety' (indicating the page number where this section is located in the Parent Manual) and briefly (one minute or so) lists the three main responses to anxiety seen in young children: avoidance, dependence, and rigid or inflexible behavior, providing the examples listed in the Parent Manual.

12. Directs the parents' attention to the next section of the Parent Manual, 'What are CBT and The Taming Sneaky Fears Program' (indicating the page number where this section is located in the Parent Manual) and:

  - Provides a brief definition of what traditional CBT is: a short-term treatment and best practice for the treatment of anxiety disorders in children over age eight years, adolescents, and adults.
  - Using Fig. 2 (asking parents to also focus on Fig. 2) and some of the text provided in the 'What are CBT and The Taming Sneaky Fears Program' section of the Parent Manual, indicates that in traditional CBT, the therapist helps the older child, adolescent, or adult to:
    - Recognize that thoughts, feelings, and behaviors are all inter-related (CBT cognitive triangle). When a situation happens, they cannot change the situation because it has already happened. What they can control is what they make of the situation (i.e., the thought they generate) and this, in turn, will affect how they feel and what they do.
    - Carefully analyze the automatic thought that comes to mind when a given situation happens and figure out whether the thought is accurate (versus inaccurate or cognitive distortion) and helpful (versus unhelpful or generating a negative emotion).
    - Challenge automatic, inaccurate, and unhelpful thoughts and replace them with thoughts that are more accurate and more helpful (this, in turn, positively affects how they feel and what they do).

  - Explains that the aforementioned concepts of traditional CBT are too cognitively sophisticated and difficult for four- to seven-year-old children to grasp and so the Taming Sneaky Fears program:
    - Uses terminology to render complex and abstracts concepts of traditional CBT more concrete and easier to understand for young children.
    - Takes a stepwise approach to teach four- to seven-year-old children complex concepts, skills, and strategies traditionally used in CBT, and adapts them to the cognitive needs of young children.

  - Uses Fig. 3 to highlight how the Taming Sneaky Fears program overlaps with traditional CBT (as was done earlier in the Introduction Session), while pointing out that in the Taming Sneaky Fears program:
    - Anxiety is *externalized* and as others have done (e.g., Huebner, 2006), children and parents are encouraged to think of anxiety, worries, and fears as unwanted visitors that the children and parents are tired of hosting, separate entities with their own names (rather than an integral and unchangeable part of the children).
    - *Sneaky Fears* refer to these unwanted visitors—these fears or worries that keep children from doing the things they want and/or need to do.
    - In the child group sessions, Sneaky Fears are made concrete by using two jackal puppets (to match the two annoying jackals that portray Sneaky Fears in the children's story and companion workbook, *Taming Sneaky*

Fears—Leo the Lion's story of bravery & Inside Leo's den: The workbook (Benoit & Monga, 2018a, b).[4] These two annoying Sneaky Fears continuously cause problems for the main story character, Leo the Lion, by appearing throughout the story and playing Tricks on Leo's brain by putting thoughts in Leo's brain that make Leo feel nervous and scared.

- Externalizing anxiety in this way sets the stage for children to be able to exert control over it, for example, children can learn to talk back to Sneaky Fears and tell their Sneaky Fears to leave them alone and quit bothering them.
- Through the program, children learn, just like Leo the Lion and his friend Ellie the Elephant learn in the story:
    (i) How to Be a Feeling Catcher (by using a Body Scan to figure out what they are feeling and by using the Feeling Thermometer to figure out how intense the feeling is).
    (ii) How to Be the Boss of My Body (by using the relaxation strategies: Spaghetti Arms and Toes, Balloon Breathing, and Imagery).
    (iii) How to Be a Trick Catcher (to catch the three Tricks Sneaky Fears that play on their brain: Not Telling the Truth, Exaggerating, and Only Showing the Bad Things).
    (iv) How to Be the Boss of My Brain (by using the Stop sign and the Trick Stoppers: Ignore Sneaky Fears, Think Brave Thoughts, and Talk to an Adult).
    (v) How to Climb Bravery Ladders (to overcome fears and show brave behavior).

13. Directs the parents' attention to the next section of the Parent Manual, 'What to Do to Help' and Fig. 4 (while indicating the page numbers where this section and Fig. 4 are located in the Parent Manual) and mentions that:

- The What to Do to Help list, which will be revisited regularly throughout the program, provides a summary of what parents can do to help their young anxious children.
- In today's Introduction Session, the focus is on the first two items of the list:
    - Make healthy lifestyle choices (the parent group therapist reads with the parents what is described in this section of the Parent Manual).

---

[4]The lead parent group therapist shows the parents a copy of the *Taming Sneaky Fears—Leo the Lion's story of bravery & Inside Leo's den: The workbook* (Benoit & Monga, 2018a, b; either original or translated version, depending on which language is used to deliver the program), provides a brief summary of the story plot, and indicates that the children will work on their own copy of the workbook section of the book, which they will take home with them at the last session. The lead child group therapist also mentions that there are more drawings to complete in the workbook than the children will have time to do in their group sessions, so parents are encouraged to help their children complete, after the group sessions are over, the sections of the workbook that could not be completed during the children's group sessions.

  – Brave moments and effective praise (the parent group therapist reads with the parents what is described in the corresponding section of the Parent Manual, emphasizing that:
      (i) Each child has temperamental or personality traits or characteristics that parents need to take into account when providing *effective praise*. For example, some children like their parents to be effusive, give high fives and two thumbs up, and other excited displays of approval when giving praise. Other children, and in fact, most children who are shy and socially anxious (for example, children with selective mutism and/or social anxiety disorder[5]), do not like overt and gushing praise as it often makes them feel that they are being put in the spotlight. Instead, they often prefer a much toned down or subtle style of praising. Parents know their children better than anyone else. So they are in the best position to *determine what style of praising suits their children's temperamental or personality traits the best*.
      (ii) As seen in the section on 'Introduction Session Tasks,' parents are asked to keep track of brave moments in their children before the next session, write down what behavior was a brave moment, and what the parent said and did as effective praise.

14. Continues to list the Introduction Session Tasks, including reading Chaps. 1–4 from Dr. Manassis' book, *Keys to parenting your anxious child* and writing down any questions for the next group session.
15. If time allows, invites parents to ask questions (if time does not allow, then asks parents to bring up questions they might have at subsequent sessions).
16. Thanks the parents for their attention, says that today's Introduction Session is over, asks the parents to remove their name tags and place them on the table, and invites them to return with their children for the next session (if a parent brings the snack for the next session, the parent group therapist reminds that parent to bring the snack).

---

[5]If children with selective mutism and/or social anxiety disorder participate in the group sessions, the parent group therapists emphasize this point.

References

Benoit, D., & Monga, S. (2018a). *Apprivoiser les Peurs-pas-fines—L'histoire de bravoure de Léo le lionceau & Dans la tanière de Léo: Le cahier de travail*. Victoria, British Columbia: FriesenPress.

Benoit, D., & Monga, S. (2018b). *Taming Sneaky Fears—Leo the Lion's story of bravery and Inside Leo's den: The workbook*. Victoria, British Columbia: FriesenPress.

Huebner, D. (2006). *What to do when you worry too much—A kid's guide to overcoming anxiety*. Washington, DC: Magination Press.

Manassis, K. (2008). *Keys to parenting your anxious child* (2nd ed.). Hauppauge, NY: Barron's Educational Series.

Chapter 8
The Taming Sneaky Fears Program: How to Be a Feeling Catcher and the Boss of My Body

8.1 Overview and Rationale

Many young children are not aware of the physical sensations associated with different feelings and for many young children the concepts of feeling recognition and management can be quite foreign. Given, however, that feeling recognition and management are central components of Cognitive Behavior Therapy (CBT) and essential skills for young anxious children to master, the first parent session (P-Session 1) and three child sessions (C-Sessions 1, 2, and 5) of the Taming Sneaky Fears program are devoted entirely to these concepts and they are revisited regularly throughout the program. Without a solid understanding and mastery of these concepts and associated skills, young anxious children often struggle with the other components of the Taming Sneaky Fears program.

Parents of young children occasionally comment that it is easier for them to manage various situations when their children can verbalize that they are feeling anxious or afraid rather than 'act up' because they cannot recognize or describe that they are, in fact, feeling anxious or afraid. Therefore, through the feeling recognition component of the Taming Sneaky Fears program (or How to Be a Feeling Catcher), parents and children learn a common language to use when talking about feelings.

The concept of becoming a Feeling Catcher helps therapists and parents explain to young children how to recognize (or 'catch') the physical clues their bodies give to signal different feelings. To become Feeling Catchers, children learn to use the Body Scan (in C-Sessions 1 and 2) and the Feeling Thermometer (in C-Session 5). In C-Sessions 1 and 2, children also learn to use three relaxation strategies to manage anxiety: Spaghetti Arms and Toes (progressive muscle relaxation), Balloon Breathing (controlled or diaphragmatic breathing), and Imagery. Children practice these relaxation strategies at the beginning of each subsequent C-Session under the

© Springer Nature Switzerland AG 2018
S. Monga and D. Benoit, *Assessing and Treating Anxiety Disorders in Young Children*, https://doi.org/10.1007/978-3-030-04939-3_8

close supervision of the child group therapists who ensure that the children use the correct techniques. In addition, parents are asked to practice each relaxation strategy at home for at least five minutes twice a day, every day, when the children are calm and relaxed and do not need the relaxation strategy, while ensuring that the children use the correct techniques. Parents and children learn that practicing each relaxation strategy correctly twice a day, every day, when calm and relaxed, allows children to master each strategy, which increases the likelihood that the strategies will work when they are needed.

8.2   Step-by-Step Guidelines to Implement Part 1 of Session 1

8.2.1   For All Parent and Child Group Therapists

8.2.1.1   During the Week Preceding Session 1

Ideally, at some point during the week preceding Session 1 (and practically, this is often done at the end of the Introduction Session), all parent group therapists meet together (if there is more than one parent group therapist) to determine which materials each parent group therapist is in charge of covering during Session 1. Similarly, the child group therapists meet to assign which specific roles each child group therapist is responsible for playing during Session 1.

All parent group and child group therapists ensure they become familiar with the materials to be covered during Session 1.

8.2.1.2   Approximately 20 minutes Prior to Start of Session 1

All parent group therapists and child group therapists meet for approximately 20 minutes (or more as needed) prior to the start of Session 1 to briefly review which child-parent dyads are expected to require assistance with the separation, which children have food allergies, intolerances, or special dietary needs/requests, and which (if any) families have cancelled Session 1.

The parent group therapists ensure that all the materials needed for P-Session 1 are available (from the list provided in Table 6.3).

Similarly, the child group therapists ensure that all the materials needed for C-Session 1 are available (from the list provided in Table 6.3).

Table 8.1   Outline of P-Session 1 (excerpt from Table 6.4)

Session[a]	Parent group	
	Minutes	
1	5	Introduction of children
	5	Debrief around separation
	10	Brave moments and effective praise

	30	How to be a Feeling Catcher
		  • Body Scan
		  • Feeling Thermometer
		How to Be the Boss of My Body
		  • Spaghetti Arms and Toes
		  • Balloon Breathing
		  • Imagery

	<1	Wrap up

[a]45- to 50-minute session; <: less than

8.2.1.3   At the Start of Session 1

At least two child and/or parent group therapists go to the waiting area to greet all parents and children and bring them to the child group room where the other child and/or parent group therapists are already waiting.[1]

As seen in Tables 8.1 and 8.2, part one of Session 1 (introduction of children) takes approximately five minutes to complete. It begins when all parents and children have entered the child group room where all the parent and child group therapists are present. One of the child group therapists takes the lead and:

1. Welcomes parents and children and invites them to sit down and make themselves comfortable.
2. Introduces all child and parent group therapists (or alternatively, the therapists can introduce themselves).
3. Has a list of each child's first name on stick-on name tags (one for each child), reads each name out loud while asking the children to identify themselves, approaches the children, asks their permission to put the stick-on name tag on their shirt or top, then asks them how old they are and what grade they are in. If verbal responses from the children are not forthcoming, non-verbal responses are encouraged, for example, asking the child to use their fingers to show how old they are, or to nod, etc. The child group therapist gives each child a few seconds to respond verbally before moving on to asking for a non-verbal response and after a few further seconds, if the children do not respond verbally or non-verbally, their parents are asked to provide the information.

---

[1]If parents are in charge of bringing the snacks for the child group sessions, it is typically at that moment that the parent who brings the snack for Session 1 gives the snack to one of the child group therapists.

Table 8.2 Outline of C-Session 1 (excerpt from Table 6.4)

Session[a]	Child group	
	Minutes	
1	5	Introduction of children
	10	Circle Time and Story Time—Chap. 1 of the children's story[b] Meet Leo the Lion and discussion of story
	5	Purpose, rules, and name of the group
	15	How to be a Feeling Catcher • Body Scans for happy and mad/angry How to Be the Boss of My Body • Spaghetti Arms and Toes
	10	Craft Time
	5	Snack Time
	<1	Wrap up—one child therapist goes to parent room to signal end of session

[a]45- to 50-minute session; [b]Children's story section of *Taming Sneaky Fears—Leo the Lion's story of bravery & Inside Leo's den: The workbook* (Benoit & Monga 2018a, b); <: less than

Developing rapport and engaging the children at the start of Session 1 facilitates the separation from the caregiver later on in the session. The child group therapists encourage verbal and non-verbal participation throughout this and all other parts of C-Session 1.

4. After all the children are introduced, the lead child group therapist says, "It's story time." This is the signal for another child group therapist to bring the container of puppets to a corner of the room, away from the door (through which parents and parent group therapists will exit), while ushering the children together towards the puppets and asking each child to choose a puppet.[2] During this time, the parent group therapists quickly, but calmly, usher the parents out of the child group room. As needed, the parent group therapists actively assist parents to leave and remind them of the instructions provided during the Introduction Session, i.e., smile, look calm and in control, and leave promptly so as to not prolong the separation and increase the children's anxiety. The child group therapists are ready and able to gently restrain or console children struggling with the separation.

Session 1 continues in the parent group room for the rest of P-Session 1 (described in Sect. 8.3.1) and in the same child group room for C-Session 1 (described in Sect. 8.4.1). This chapter also includes step-by-step guidelines to implement C-Session 2 (Sect. 8.5.1) and C-Session 5 (Sect. 8.6.1) as all these child group sessions focus on the concepts of feeling recognition and management.

---

[2]The list of puppets the children can use and the puppets reserved for the child group therapists is provided in Sect. 6.3.3.2.

8.3 Step-by-Step Guidelines to Implement P-Session 1

8.3.1 Part One of P-Session 1

After the parents depart the child group room and enter the parent group room, the components of P-Session 1 dealing exclusively with the parents start. As seen in Table 8.1, the first part of P-Session 1 (introduction of children) was completed in about five minutes (as described in the previous sections) and there are four additional parts for parent group therapists to complete in P-Session 1.

8.3.2 Part Two of P-Session 1

As the parents enter the parent group room in P-Session 1 and each subsequent P-Session, one of the parent group therapists welcomes the parents and invites them to take their name tag from the table and put it on as they make themselves comfortable.

If parents are in charge of bringing the snack at each session, the lead parent group therapist thanks the parent who brought the snack for the child group session today and reminds the parents of which parent is in charge of bringing the children's snack for the next session.

The lead parent group therapist then facilitates part two of P-Session 1 (debrief around separation), which could take approximately five minutes to complete. If some children and/or parents struggled with the separation, the lead parent group therapist could ask all parents how they think the separation went. Oftentimes, parents report that their children reacted as expected. The lead parent group therapist reminds the parents that the child group therapists are experienced in helping young children manage separation anxiety and will come and get parents to assist only if necessary, which is a rare occurrence. However, if no children or parents had any difficulty with the separation, the parent group therapist could briefly comment on how well the separation went and proceed with the program.

8.3.3 Part Three of P-Session 1

Part three of P-Session 1 (brave moments and effective praise) takes approximately ten minutes to complete and uses the following protocol, which is used at most subsequent P-Sessions (except P-Sessions 4 and 8). The parent group therapists ask parents to volunteer examples of brave moments they noticed in their children since the previous session and how they provided effective praise. The parent group therapists encourage parent engagement by:

1. Inviting supportive comments from other parents on what the parents volunteering examples did well when providing effective praise and what they could have done differently to make the praise even more effective.
2. Asking parents to review the three main characteristics of effective praise (i.e., start praise with a 'You' statement, focus on *specific behavior* displayed by the child, provide praise *as soon as possible* after the display of brave behavior).
3. Asking parents to explain the rationale for identifying brave moments and providing effective praise (i.e., the more one pays attention to a behavior, the more often that behavior is likely to be repeated).

Throughout this part, the parent group therapists actively provide constructive feedback to the parents who volunteer examples and comments. The parent group therapists remind the parents that focusing on brave moments and providing effective praise are tasks to do throughout the program (and ideally, would continue even after the Taming Sneaky Fears program is completed).

8.3.4 Part Four of P-Session 1

Part four of P-Session 1 (How to Be a Feeling Catcher and How to Be the Boss of My Body) is content heavy, takes approximately 30 minutes to complete, and consists of providing psychoeducation on feeling identification (or How to Be a Feeling Catcher by doing a Body Scan and using the Feeling Thermometer) and management (or How to Be the Boss of My Body by using the three relaxation strategies: Spaghetti Arms and Toes, Balloon Breathing, and Imagery). The parent group therapists need to carefully pace themselves and their rate of delivery of information in this part of P-Session 1 to ensure that they have enough time to cover all the materials.[3]

8.3.4.1 Introduction

To begin part four of P-Session 1 the parent group therapist leading this portion:

1. Uses the laminated copy of Fig. 3 from the Parent Manual[4] illustrating the overlap between traditional CBT and the Taming Sneaky Fears program to emphasize that during today's parent session the focus is on the 'Feeling' component of the cognitive triangle, so in today's session parents learn:

    a. How to Be a Feeling Catcher by doing a Body Scan (the lead parent group therapist indicates that the children learn about Body Scans during today's

---

[3]If the parent group therapists do not have enough time to deliver all the information that is planned in P-Session 1, we recommend covering the material that was not covered in P-Session 1 at the beginning of P-Session 2, but be aware that P-Session 2 is also content heavy, so it is best for the parent group therapists to carefully pace themselves.

[4]The Parent Manual is provided as one of the Supplementary Materials in Chap. 6.

session and the next session) and using the Feeling Thermometer (the lead parent group therapist indicates that the children learn about the Feeling Thermometer in Session 5 and asks parents to refrain from using the term Feeling Thermometer until then).

b. How to Be the Boss of My Body by doing relaxation strategies: Spaghetti Arms and Toes (progressive muscle relaxation), Balloon Breathing (controlled or diaphragmatic breathing), and Imagery; the lead parent group therapist indicates that the children learn about Spaghetti Arms and Toes during today's session and learn about Balloon Breathing and Imagery during the next session, and asks parents to refrain from using the terms Balloon Breathing and Imagery until the next session).

2. Shows the two children's workbooks (the workbook section of *Taming Sneaky Fears—Leo the Lion's story of bravery & Inside Leo's den: The workbook* (Benoit & Monga 2018a, b) and the Supplementary Child Workbook[5]) and points out the crafts the children are asked to do today to consolidate the concepts they are learning in their session today: How to Be a Feeling Catcher by doing a Body Scan for happy and one for mad or angry, and How to Be the Boss of My Body by doing Spaghetti Arms and Toes. The lead parent group therapist mentions that:

a. The parents do not have the children's workbooks in their possession, as these are kept with the child group therapists until Session 8 ('graduation') when the two children's workbooks are given to the children to take home with them.

b. The workbook section of *Taming Sneaky Fears—Leo the Lion's story of bravery & Inside Leo's den: The workbook* (Benoit & Monga 2018a, b) contains more activities the children could do than time allows in the child group sessions, so at the end of the group program, parents could complete these additional activities with the children to help them further integrate the concepts they have learned during the group sessions.

3. Mentions that the children will do Body Scans for nervous or scared and shy at the next session (when they also learn about Balloon Breathing and Imagery).

4. Reminds parents they can use the following terminology with the children after today's session: How to Be a Feeling Catcher by doing a Body Scan and How to Be the Boss of My Body by doing Spaghetti Arms and Toes.

5. Reminds parents to refrain from using terminology children have not covered yet in their sessions (e.g., Balloon Breathing, Imagery, the Feeling Thermometer, Sneaky Fears) and that the parent group therapists will inform them of when the children are introduced to the various new terminology.

---

[5]The Supplementary Child Workbook is provided as one of the Supplementary Materials in Chap. 6.

8.3.4.2   How to Be a Feeling Catcher

The parent group therapist leading this portion:

1. Asks the parents to go to Session 1 in their Parent Manual (and points to the page number).
2. Encourages parents to follow along as the therapist covers the following materials about How to Be a Feeling Catcher and do a Body Scan in the Parent Manual:

   a. Feelings do not happen somewhere in one's head or mind. They happen somewhere in one's body, i.e., they are bodily sensations:
      i.   When young children feel *nervous*, they feel it somewhere in their bodies (i.e., fast/pounding heart beat, breathing fast or trouble catching breath, throat tightening, tummy ache, nausea, tingling or numbing sensations in fingers or toes, shaking, feeling hot or cold, sweating, tight and sore muscles, etc.).
      ii. When they feel *sad*, they also feel this emotion somewhere in their bodies (i.e., teary eyes, lump in throat, like a puddle in their tummy, etc.).
      iii. When they feel *angry*, they feel it in their bodies as well (i.e., clenched teeth and jaw, tense muscles, scowl on face, red face, clenched fists, etc.).

   b. The body sensations and manifestations (or physical appearance) associated with feeling happy are different from the body sensations and manifestations associated with feeling sad, nervous or scared, angry or mad, or shy. In fact, the cluster of *body sensations and manifestations associated with each emotion is unique to that specific emotion*. For example, and as pointed out in the Parent Manual, if a child (or adult) has a scowl on his red face, clenched teeth, clenched fists, and makes growling sounds, one is not likely to think that that person feels happy. One is likely to think that that person feels angry.

   c. By showing children How to Be a Feeling Catcher and 'catch' the physical clues their bodies give to signal different feelings, the Taming Sneaky Fears program helps children to:
      i.   Recognize *where they feel each emotion in their body* (the Body Scan exercises and charades help children accomplish this).
      ii. Recognize that *each emotion feels different in different parts of the body*.

   d. When children learn to be Feeling Catchers and figure out clues their bodies give when feeling a specific emotion, they are better able to identify what they feel and communicate that feeling to their parents or others around them. It becomes easier for parents and other adults to help children identify what they feel by doing a Body Scan (or charade).

   e. In the child group, as children do their drawings of a Body Scan for each emotion [using the body outlines provided in the relevant sections of the workbook section of *Taming Sneaky Fears—Leo's story of bravery & Inside Leo's Den: The workbook* (Benoit & Monga 2018a, b)], they start to realize that nervous or scared feels different in different parts of the body compared to happy, angry or mad, sad, etc.

3. Suggests that parents and children practice doing Body Scans (and/or charades) for different feelings at home (using the 'How to Do a Body Scan' section and Figs. 10–13 of the Parent Manual). This will help parents and children have a common language to express and understand what the children are feeling at different times. For example, when a child complains of a sore tummy in the morning just before it is time to leave for school, the parent could help the child be a Feeling Catcher by doing a quick (or more extensive, as needed) Body Scan of how each part of the child's body feels and thereby 'catch' the emotion the child feels, e.g., nervous and scared about the show and share activity that is coming up at school that day.

4. Recommends, as mentioned in item 3 of the What to Do to Help list (Fig. 4 of the Parent Manual), that parents practice doing Body Scans (or charades) with their children to help them master the skill of being a Feeling Catcher to identify what emotion their body is feeling, otherwise it is difficult to move forward with the other strategies utilized in this program. If children have trouble being a Feeling Catcher, doing Body Scans, and recognizing what they feel, the parents might wish to spend extra time completing additional Body Scans and/or charades, especially involving the feelings nervous or scared and shy.

8.3.4.3 How to Do a Body Scan

The parent group therapist leading this portion:

1. Asks the parents to go to the section of the Parent Manual on How to Do a Body Scan (and points out the page number).

2. Shows the parents Fig. 6 of the Parent Manual (Body Scan) then shows parents the four Body Scans (Figs. 10–13 of the Parent Manual) that parents are asked to complete with their young children after today's session and after the next session (the Body Scans to complete after today's session are for happy and mad or angry; the Body Scans to complete after the next session are for nervous or scared and shy).

3. Suggests to parents that they could help their children review what they have learned in the child group sessions 1 and 2 by asking them to show and/or tell the parents (or other family members) How to Be a Feeling Catcher and do a Body Scan (this way, the parents can also make sure that the children are mastering this skill).

4. Mentions that some parents find that doing charades is a fun way (and sometimes more helpful than doing Body Scans) for their young children to understand the concept of how their body feels and looks when experiencing a specific emotion.

5. Directs the parents' attention to the script to help young children do a Body Scan (and points out the appropriate page in the Parent Manual). The therapist does not read verbatim what is written in this section, but only points out to the parents that the script includes examples of questions parents could ask as they do Body Scans with their young children. Essentially, to do a Body Scan, parents help their

children figure out how each part of the child's body feels and looks, starting at the top of the child's body (head and face), then focusing on shoulders, neck and throat, heart, lungs/breathing, tummy, muscles, all the way down to the child's extremities.

6. Directs the parents' attention to the summary of examples of body sensations and manifestations associated with different emotions (and points out the page number on which this information is found in the Parent Manual); the therapist does not read this section verbatim, but only mentions to parents that they could refer to that section as needed when they are doing Body Scans with their young children.

8.3.4.4   The Feeling Thermometer

The parent group therapist leading this portion:

1. Asks the parents to go to the section of the Parent Manual on the Feeling Thermometer (and points out the page number where this information is found).
2. Reminds parents that children learn about the Feeling Thermometer only in Session 5 (so refrain from using this terminology until then).
3. Uses a laminated copy of the Feeling Thermometer (Fig. 8 of the Parent Manual) to explain that feelings have different intensities, going from a 0 to a 10, and these feeling intensities are associated with different body sensations. For example:

   a. One can feel a little bit scared (in the children's story that is read to the children, Ellie the Elephant describes that when her cousin, Eleanor the Elephant, jumps out from behind a chair and says "boo," that is just a little scary, like a 1 or 2 on the Feeling Thermometer); the associated body sensations might be a little skip of her heart beat.
   b. One can feel moderately nervous or scared, like a 4 or 5 on the Feeling Thermometer; the associated body sensations would be more intense and probably include eyes open big and wide, eyebrows arched up, no smile, throat feeling tight and closed up, heart knocking in chest, choppy breathing, butterflies in the stomach or sore tummy, and/or stiff muscles.
   c. One can feel the most nervous or scared possible, like a 9 or 10 on the Feeling Thermometer; the associated body sensations would be even more intense than those described when at a 4 or 5 on the Feeling Thermometer and resemble an intense panic attack.

4. Uses the laminated copy of the Feeling Thermometer to point out that when a child feels a negative emotion at a 5 or higher on the Feeling Thermometer:

   a. The emotion is too intense and overwhelming.
   b. There is no point in trying to reason with a child who is distressed at a 5 or above on the Feeling Thermometer because the child is too distressed and cannot think clearly.

    c. It is time to Be the Boss of My Body and make the Feeling Thermometer go down to a more manageable level, i.e., a 1 or a 2, by using the relaxation strategies (Spaghetti Arms and Toes, Balloon Breathing, and Imagery).

5. Directs the parents' attention to the script on How to Use the Feeling Thermometer (and points out the page number where this information can be found in the Parent Manual); the parent group therapist does not read this information verbatim, but only mentions to the parents that they could use that script if they wish when showing their young children how to use the Feeling Thermometer (after Session 5).

6. Recommends, as mentioned in item 4 of the What to Do to Help list (Fig. 4 of the Parent Manual), that parents practice using the Feeling Thermometer with their children, but only after Session 5 (i.e., after the children learn about the Feeling Thermometer during the group).

8.3.4.5   How to Be the Boss of My Body

The parent group therapist leading this portion:

1. Asks the parents to go to the section of the Parent Manual on How to Be the Boss of My Body (and points out the page number where this information is found).

2. Points out to the parents that during today's session, we, as adults, practice each of the relaxation strategies (but the children learn only Spaghetti Arms and Toes today).

3. Mentions that after today's session (as described in the Session 1 Tasks section of the Parent Manual), we ask that parents help their children practice Spaghetti Arms and Toes for at least five minutes, twice a day, every day, when the children are calm and do not need relaxation strategies, in order to master the strategy so that it will work when the children need it (without this intensive daily practice, it is unlikely that this and any other relaxation strategy would work when needed); recommends to parents to use the practice chart provided for the various strategies (Figs. 14–16 of the Parent Manual).

Spaghetti Arms and Toes

The parent group therapist leading this portion:

1. Tells the parents that we are going to practice Spaghetti Arms and Toes using the script that is used with the children in their session today.

2. Asks the parents to sit comfortably on their chair, place their feet flat on the floor and hold their arms loosely down to their sides as they close their eyes and follow directions; the lead parent group therapist proceeds to read out loud the entire script for Spaghetti Arms and Toes (from the Parent Manual); the parent group therapist uses a lively voice as if speaking to the young children in the child group room.

3. After doing Spaghetti Arms and Toes, reminds the parents that the children are likely to require their active help at first to practice this relaxation strategy to ensure that the children are using the proper technique; the goal is to have the children eventually be skilled enough in doing this relaxation strategy that parental assistance is no longer needed.
4. Mentions to the parents that after children are skilled at using the correct techniques, they might not need to lie down to do Spaghetti Arms and Toes; they might only need to pretend to squeeze a lemon tightly as they tighten their whole body (while sitting, standing, or lying down) to feel the benefit.

Balloon Breathing

The parent group therapist leading this portion:

1. Tells the parents that we are now going to practice Balloon Breathing during our group session, using the script that will be used with the children in their next session.
2. Reminds the parents not to ask children to 'take a deep breath' when doing Balloon Breathing as 'taking a deep breath' would be more akin to hyperventilating, which typically worsens anxiety symptoms.
3. Demonstrates the correct technique by sitting sideways so the parents can see clearly the demonstration:
   a. Places one hand on the chest and one hand between the belly button and rib cage (often times, the parents will do the same and the lead parent group therapist encourages this).
   b. Explains that when doing Balloon Breathing (diaphragmatic breathing), only the hand on the abdomen moves: up when one breathes in and down when one breathes out; the hand on the chest remains completely immobile, i.e., the chest and shoulders are relaxed and do not move at all when doing Balloon Breathing.
   c. Proceeds to demonstrate four or five Balloon Breaths using the correct technique.
4. Asks the parents to sit comfortably on their chair, place their feet flat on the floor and place one hand on their chest and one hand between their belly button and rib cage as they close their eyes and follow directions (from the script that the parent group therapist reads out loud).
5. Reads out loud the entire script for Balloon Breathing (from the Parent Manual) using a calm and relaxing voice (loud enough to be heard easily by all parents).
6. Asks the parents to slowly breathe in through the nose and slowly breathe out through the mouth, as if blowing a birthday candle; when breathing out, a 'mantra' could be used, such as 'calm down,' 'relax,' or 'you're safe.'
7. Asks the parents to practice doing ten Balloon Breaths slowly as the parent group therapists provide individual feedback to the parents on their technique.

8. Suggests that the parents practice in front of a mirror at home (directly facing the mirror or sitting sideways so the hands on the chest and abdomen are seen clearly) if they have trouble using the proper technique.
9. After doing Balloon Breathing, reminds the parents that the children are likely to require their active help at first when practicing this relaxation strategy to ensure that the children are using the correct technique; the goal is to have the children eventually be skilled enough in doing this relaxation strategy that parental assistance is no longer needed; also, after the children master the proper technique, they will no longer need to place a hand on their chest and a hand on their abdomen, i.e., they will be able to use Balloon Breathing discretely in all settings, whether they are sitting, standing, or lying down.

Balloon Breathing and Imagery Together

The parent group therapist leading this portion:

1. Tells the parents we are going to practice doing Imagery and Balloon Breathing together in the parent group today, and mentions that the children are told in their group that using these two relaxation strategies together works even better than using each of these relaxation strategies on its own.
2. Tells the parents that the parent group therapist will read the script that will be used with the children at their next session (and points at where this script is located in the Parent Manual).
3. Asks the parents to close their eyes and do Balloon Breathing as they immerse themselves in what is being said in the Imagery script.
4. After the Imagery script is read, reviews how the Imagery script incorporates sensations from all senses.
5. Encourages the parents to have their children draw a picture of their own safe and calm place that incorporates all the senses (sight, sound/hearing, smell, taste, and touch or feel on skin); emphasizes drawing a *calm and safe* place, not a happy place (happy involves a certain degree of excitement and what we want the children to do when doing Imagery is relax, not get excited); drawing a picture of their calm and safe place makes it easier for children to visualize it when doing Imagery and for parents to help their children do Imagery effectively.

8.3.4.6   Conclusions

The parent group therapist leading this part:

1. Emphasizes the importance of making sure the children use the correct techniques when practicing each of the relaxation strategies at home.
2. Reiterates that young children typically need a lot of practice to master each relaxation strategy to cope with shyness, fear, anxiety, and other negative emotion, and even worries.

3. Recommends, as mentioned in item 5 of the What to Do to Help list (Fig. 4 of the Parent Manual), that parents practice with their children Spaghetti Arms and Toes (and starting after next session each of the three relaxation strategies), twice a day, every day, for at least five minutes each time, using the correct technique, when the children do not need the strategies, i.e., when they are calm and relaxed.

4. Reminds the parents that unless young children practice the relaxation strategies often, and when their bodies are calm and relaxed (to master the strategies), the relaxation strategies are not likely to work when needed.

5. Reminds the parents that after Session 5, they will help their children figure out when to use Spaghetti Arms and Toes, Balloon Breathing, and Imagery, i.e., when they are at a 5 or above on the Feeling Thermometer for shy, nervous or scared, or angry (or other negative emotion), but for all the sessions until then, the children are encouraged to learn to master the proper technique for each relaxation strategy.

6. Mentions that it is often challenging to get young children to practice as long and as often as needed; encourages the parents to be creative in how to motivate their children to practice every day (and asks for the parents' suggestions on how to encourage young children to practice as often as needed; as indicated in the Parent Manual, some parents make practicing the relaxation strategies an every day part of their children's regular schedule and routine, just like brushing teeth morning and night is part of the routine and has to be done. Making the practice of relaxation strategies part of the regular, daily routine might be the most effective strategy to get children to practice as often as needed. Using reward systems to help motivate young children to add the practice of relaxation strategies to their regular routine often proves helpful. Other parents find that getting their children to teach family members how to do relaxation or having everyone in the family practice the relaxation strategies at the same time can be motivating).

The lead parent group therapist then directs the parents' attention to the Parent Session 1 Tasks (and points out the page number where this section is located in the Parent Manual) and briefly reviews the task items that were not already discussed during today's session.

8.3.5   Part Five of P-Session 1

Part five of P-Session 1 (wrap up) takes 30–60 seconds to complete and is the same for all subsequent sessions. It starts when one of the child group therapists knocks at the door and enters the parent group room to provide a ten-second summary of the topic covered during the child session that day. As soon as the child group therapist departs, the lead parent therapist thanks the parents for their attention and cooperation today, wishes them well, and reminds them:

1. That the child group therapist coming in is the signal for the parent group session to end promptly as the children are ready to be picked up.

2. To remove their name tags and place them on the table as these are re-used at each session.
3. To go to the children's group room to pick up their children (one of the parent group therapists might lead the way to the child group room to remind parents of its location).

8.4 Step-by-Step Guidelines to Implement C-Session 1

Before C-Session 1 begins, the child group therapists decide amongst themselves who is responsible for the various tasks of the session and ensure that all the materials needed for C-Session 1 are available (from the list provided in Table 6.3). Just as C-Session 1 is about to start, and as described in Sect. 8.2.1.3, at least two child group and/or parent group therapists go to the waiting area, greet parents and children, and bring them to the child group room (the other child group and parent group therapists are already in the child group room). As seen in Table 8.2, C-Session 1 is divided into seven parts.

8.4.1 Part One of C-Session 1

The role of the child group therapists in part one of C-Session 1 (introduction of children) is described in Sect. 8.2.1.3.

8.4.2 Part Two of C-Session 1

Part two of C-Session 1 (Circle Time, Story Time, and discussion of story) takes about ten minutes to complete and begins when the child group therapist leading this portion of the session directs the children to sit in a semi circle with the puppet they chose, while the other child group therapists sit interspersed amongst the children. Before reading the story, the lead child group therapist spends a minute re-introducing everyone. Pretending to remember everyone's name can be a fun way to re-engage the children. The child group therapist taking the lead for reading the story encourages engagement by asking the children if they like stories. Usually, some children raise their hands. If no children respond, one of the other child group therapists may state that they enjoy stories.

One child group therapist reads Story Chap. 1 in the children's story section of *Taming Sneaky Fears—Leo the Lion's story of bravery & Inside Leo's den: The workbook* (Benoit & Monga 2018a, b) with a lively and engaging voice and animated facial expressions while showing the illustrations.

8.4.2.1 Story Discussion

In Story Chap. 1, the main story character, Leo the Lion, is introduced. Leo the Lion is a small lion who is supposed to be brave because he is the "King of the Jungle." However, he does not feel brave and, in fact, he feels scared and nervous. Leo the Lion is afraid of his roar and feels too shy to make new friends. After Story Chap. 1 is read, the child group therapist leading the story discussion (two to three minutes in duration) asks if the children liked the story and allows for verbal and nonverbal responses, while actively encouraging verbal responses. If no child responds, one of the other child group therapists can answer in a positive fashion, thus modeling verbal interaction. The goals of the story discussion are to encourage the children to identify with Leo the Lion (e.g., Leo and I both feel scared and nervous), help the children begin to understand some physical signs of anxiety (e.g., my tummy hurts like Leo the Lion's when I feel nervous), and help the children begin to understand that, like Leo, they can learn How to Be the Boss of their Body.

The lead child group therapist continues the discussion and asks the children if, like Leo the Lion, they worry or feel shy, nervous, or scared sometimes. Questions could focus specifically on some of the fears and worries that the children in the group actually have as this can help children understand the purpose of the group. For example, if there are children with separation anxiety in the group, a question might focus on whether anyone feels nervous and scared about sleeping alone. If none of the children articulate any fears or worries or respond to questions, another child group therapist could respond (with child age-appropriate examples of various common childhood fears, again using examples that might specifically pertain to children in the group). And finally, the lead child group therapist asks the children if they remember what Leo the Lion learned to do in the story and awaits a response that Leo learned that he could Be the Boss of his Body and he learned to do Spaghetti Arms and Toes (if no response if forthcoming from the children, another child group therapist provides the answers).

8.4.3 Part Three of C-Session 1

As seen in Table 8.2, part three of C-Session 1 (purpose, rules, and name of the group) takes about five minutes to complete and focuses on providing the children with an explanation for the purpose of the group and having them come up with rules and a name for the group. The child group therapist leading this portion of the session:

1. Refers back to the story, pointing out how Leo the Lion is going to a Bravery Club to learn to be brave, and explains that just like Leo will be going to a Bravery Club, the children here will meet at each session to learn how to be brave.
2. Asks the children if they have a suggestion for what the name of their group could be. With more verbal groups (e.g., groups in which fewer children have either social anxiety disorder or selective mutism) a name for the group is usually

easily generated by the children themselves; however, suggestions for the name of the group could be provided to the children by the child group therapists, using variations on being or becoming brave (e.g., Leo's Bravery Group, the Tuesday Be Brave Club (if the group takes place on a Tuesday), the Puppet Bravery Club). While the lead child group therapist directs the discussion and writes the suggestions for a group name on the white board (or flip chart), the other child group therapists encourage children by providing ideas, and even encouraging socially anxious and selectively mute children to whisper a suggestion to the therapist. Once two or three group names have been generated and written down on the white board (or flip chart), the lead child group therapist further engages the children in choosing the name of their group by suggesting they vote on the name. Having the children raise their hand to vote on the name of the group allows for engagement of even socially anxious and selectively mute children. The group name that gets the most votes from the children is the 'winner' and the child group therapist who comes to the parent room at the end of the session mentions the name of the group to the parents. Additionally, the name of the group will be prominently displayed on the graduation certificate (Fig. 11.1) the child receives at C-Session 8 (graduation).

3. Asks the children for suggestions for rules for the group and spends a few minutes enlisting the children's help to come up with three to five rules for the group (e.g., take turns talking, listen, be nice (or no pushing or hurting), ask questions if you do not understand something). The final rule could be to have fun. These rules are written on the white board (or flip chart). Typically, the rules are not revisited from session to session. However, when there are disruptive children within the group, the list of rules could be pulled out and children could be reminded about the rules they helped to generate.

The puppets are returned to the container before moving on to part four.

8.4.4   Part Four of C-Session 1

Part four of C-Session 1 takes about 15 minutes to complete and teaches the children two concepts: (1) How to Be a Feeling Catcher by learning how to do a Body Scan and (2) How to Be the Boss of My Body by learning how to do Spaghetti Arms and Toes.

8.4.4.1   How to Be a Feeling Catcher

The child group therapist leading this portion of the session:

1. Explains that to be a Feeling Catcher, children look for and 'catch' the clues that their body gives that tell them they are feeling something like happy, sad, mad or angry, nervous or scared, or shy.

2. Asks the children if they can think of any feelings that Leo the Lion felt in the story (i.e., nervous or scared and mad or angry).
3. Asks how they could tell that Leo felt nervous or scared (i.e., his muscles were all stiff and hard like uncooked spaghetti and his tummy felt sore) and mad or angry (i.e., he kicked the toy and slammed the door extra hard).

8.4.4.2   How to Do a Body Scan

The child group therapist leading the discussion on Body Scans uses a large laminated picture of a genderless child body outline or draws a large child body outline on the white board (or flip chart) for this portion of the session. The children are asked to gather around the body outline and in this C-Session 1, the feelings of happy and mad or angry are discussed and Body Scans of these two feelings are completed. The lead child group therapist:

1. Begins by telling the children that today they are going to learn How to Be a Feeling Catcher and learn to 'catch' the clues within their body that tell them they are feeling a certain feeling.
2. Tells the children that in order to be a Feeling Catcher, the first thing they need to do is a Body Scan and points to the body outline.
3. Explains that in order to do a Body Scan, the children need to think about how every part of their body looks and feels when they are feeling happy (or later on mad or angry), starting with their head and going all the way down to their toes.
4. Asks the children to think about how their face, eyes, cheeks, and mouth look and feel like when they are happy (and later mad or angry). A good starting suggestion could be to ask the children if they can make a happy face as this can easily lead to a discussion of how a happy face looks. Using the script from page 16 in the Parent Manual, examples of questions could be: What does your face look like when you are happy? Is your forehead relaxed or are your eyebrows lifted? Do you have a smile or frown on your face? Are your eyes bright and shiny, or are they full of tears, or almost closed? Are your jaws all relaxed or are they all stiff? Are your cheeks all red or their usual color?
5. Draws on the large laminated body outline (or on the body outline that was drawn on the white board or flip chart) the suggestions provided by the children of what one's face looks like when feeling happy.
6. Asks the children what their shoulders, neck, and throat look and feel like when they are happy (and later mad or angry), while using the script from page 16 in the Parent Manual to ask questions such as: Are your shoulders relaxed or all stiff and raised up close to your ears? Is your neck relaxed or are the muscles in your neck so stiff that you almost have a headache? Is your throat relaxed or all tight? Do you feel a lump in your throat? Do you lose your voice?
7. Draws on the body outline the suggestions provided by the children of what one's shoulders, neck, and throat would look and feel like when feeling happy.

8. Asks the children what the insides of their body feel like when they are happy (and later mad or angry), using the script from page 16 in the Parent Manual with questions such as, does your heart beat fast or hard or it is calm and relaxed? Is your breathing calm or too fast and choppy, like it's hard to catch your breath? Do you feel butterflies in your tummy? Is your tummy sore or does your tummy feel nice and calm?

9. Draws on the body outline the suggestions provided by the children of what the inside of one's body feels like when one feels happy.

10. Asks the children what their arms, fingers, and legs look and feel like when they are happy (and later mad or angry), using the script from page 16 in the Parent Manual with questions such as, are the muscles of your body all relaxed or all stiff and hard? Are your hands and feet all calm or are they shaking? Are your hands and fingers all relaxed or are they stiff or closed in fists?

11. Draws on the body outline the suggestions provided by the children of what one's extremities would look and feel like when feeling happy.

For C-Session 1, a completed Body Scan for happy could have a smiling face, calm heart and calm breathing, and relaxed muscles while the completed Body Scan for mad or angry could have tight or squeezed eyes, furrowed eyebrows, clenched or tightly closed mouth, clenched fists, and stomping feet.

8.4.4.3 How to Be the Boss of My Body

After completing the Body Scans for happy and for mad or angry, the child group therapist leading the discussion on How to Be the Boss of My Body teaches the children the first relaxation strategy, Spaghetti Arms and Toes. Ideally, children lie down on the floor on a mat as this is more relaxing and children can isolate each muscle group more easily. However, young children could learn each strategy while sitting comfortably in their chairs. If feasible, the lights are dimmed (without making the room too dark) while completing the relaxation strategies and then the lights are turned back on. The lead child group therapist:

1. Informs the children that just like Leo the Lion in the story they are going to learn How to Be the Boss of their Body.

2. Asks if anyone knows what uncooked spaghetti looks and feels like and what cooked spaghetti looks and feels like (and ensures that the children understand that uncooked spaghetti is stiff and hard while cooked spaghetti is soft and pliable).

3. Describes that just like Leo the Lion, when they do Spaghetti Arms and Toes they learn how to make their muscles get all hard and stiff, like uncooked spaghetti noodles, and then make them all soft and wiggly, like cooked spaghetti.

The lead child group therapist then reads the Spaghetti Arms and Toes script provided in Sect. 8.4.4.4 below (which is the same script as that found in the Parent

Manual) and runs through each muscle group twice. The script for Spaghetti Arms and Toes is similar to the one found on page 55 in the workbook section of *Taming Sneaky Fears—Leo the Lions's story of bravery & Inside Leo's den: The workbook* (Benoit & Monga 2018a, b), but contains one main difference, i.e., in the group program, parents and children are encouraged to pretend squeezing the juice out of lemons when completing Spaghetti Arms and Toes (with practice, children who feel tense and nervous can simply squeeze their fists as if they are squeezing the juice out of lemons and then relax them, and get the same benefit as completing the full Spaghetti Arms and Toes script[6]).

8.4.4.4   Spaghetti Arms and Toes Script

Close your eyes so you can pay attention to how your muscles feel in your body. Let's start with your **toes** and **feet**. Point your toes and feet straight up towards the ceiling and tighten up your feet and toes as tight as they can be. Make sure your feet and toes are hard and stiff like uncooked spaghetti. Hold them really tight and count to five slowly—one, two, three, four, five. Feel how hard the muscles in your feet and toes feel. Your muscles might feel a little sore because they're so stiff. Now pretend your feet and toes are going in warm water and you can let them loosen up. Feel how nice and soft and relaxed the muscles in your feet and toes feel, just like cooked spaghetti. Your muscles feel warm and nice and relaxed.

Now lift and tighten up your **legs** and **thighs**. Make both of your legs and thighs really tight and stiff like uncooked spaghetti noodles and count to five slowly—one, two, three, four, five. Feel how hard the muscles in your legs and thighs feel. Your muscles might feel a little sore because they're so stiff. Now your legs and thighs are going in the warm water and you can let them loosen up. Feel how nice and soft and relaxed the muscles in your legs and thighs feel. Your muscles feel warm and nice and relaxed.

Now hold your **arms** and **hands** out in front of you really straight and stiff like uncooked spaghetti and squeeze your **fists** like you're squeezing lemons. Make sure your arms and hands are hard and stiff like uncooked spaghetti and you squeeze your fists as if you are squeezing the juice out of lemons. Hold everything really tight, squeeze those lemons, and count to five slowly—one, two, three, four, five. Feel how hard the muscles in your arms and hands and squeezed fists feel. Your muscles might feel a little sore because they're so stiff. Now they're going in the warm water and you can let them loosen up. Feel how nice and soft and relaxed the muscles in your arms and hands and fingers feel, just like cooked spaghetti. Your muscles feel warm and nice and relaxed.

Now scrunch up your **face** and tighten your **neck** and **shoulders** so your shoulders touch your ears. Make the muscles in your face, neck, and shoulders really stiff and

---

[6]Koeppen (1974) first described how group therapists could encourage children to squeeze their fists as if they are squeezing the juice out of lemons when doing progressive muscle relaxation. The Taming Sneaky Fears group treatment program adopted this strategy.

tight, just like uncooked spaghetti noodles, and count to five slowly—one, two, three, four, five. Feel how hard the muscles in your face, neck, and shoulders feel. The muscles in your face, neck, and shoulders might feel a little sore because they're so stiff. Now the muscles in your face, neck, and shoulders are going in the warm water and becoming loose and relaxed, just like cooked spaghetti noodles. Feel how nice and soft and relaxed the muscles in your face, neck, and shoulders feel. Your muscles feel warm and nice and relaxed.

Now make your **whole body** as stiff as one giant uncooked spaghetti, so tighten up your **toes**, **feet**, **legs** and **thighs**, tighten up your **arms** and **hands**, and squeeze your **fists**, and tighten up your whole body including your **face**, **neck**, and **shoulders** and even your **back** and **tummy**. Hold everything really stiff and count to five slowly—one, two, three, four, five. Feel how hard all of the muscles in your whole body feel—like one giant uncooked spaghetti. Your muscles might feel a little sore because they're so stiff. You might even feel your tummy is getting a little sore. Now your whole body is going into the warm water and getting really soft and wobbly. The muscles in your whole body feel warm and nice and relaxed. Doesn't that feel good?

8.4.5   Part Five of C-Session 1

As seen in Table 8.2, part five of C-Session 1 (Craft Time) takes approximately ten minutes to complete.

8.4.5.1   Craft Time—General Format for All C-Sessions

The primary purpose of Craft Time for all child group sessions is to help children internalize the concepts they learn during each session. Craft Time follows the same format at each child group session. Craft Time takes ten minutes to complete and begins when one child group therapist asks the children to come to the table to complete the craft(s). When implementing a child group using the Taming Sneaky Fears program, for the most part, children use the workbook section of *Taming Sneaky Fears—Leo the Lion's story of bravery & Inside Leo's den: The workbook* (Benoit & Monga 2018a, b). However, as detailed in subsequent chapters, children participating in a group treatment program complete additional crafts from the Supplementary Child Workbook, which is found in the Chap. 6 supplementary materials. As one of the child group therapists directs the children to the table, another child group therapist distributes the workbook(s) to each child (the workbooks will be gifted to the children as part of their graduation gift; see Chap. 11).

8.4.5.2 Specific Craft for C-Session 1

One of the child group therapists leads the craft activity by explaining what is required and demonstrating what to draw on the white board (or flip chart) as needed. The child group therapists distribute the two workbooks to the children and instruct them to write their name on the first inside page of *Taming Sneaky Fears—Leo the Lion's story of bravery & Inside Leo's den: The workbook* (Benoit & Monga 2018a, b) and on the cover page of the Supplementary Child Workbook in the space provided for child's name. The child group therapists may need to help younger children write their name. At the beginning of Craft Time for all subsequent C-Sessions, the child group therapists distribute the required workbook(s) and ensure the children use the correct page(s) of each workbook. During Craft Time at C-Session 1, the children complete three drawings:

1. The first drawing is found on page 53 in the workbook section of *Taming Sneaky Fears—Leo the Lion's story of bravery & Inside Leo's den: The workbook* (Benoit & Monga 2018a, b). Children draw their own Body Scan for happy using the large body outline drawn earlier in the group as a template. The child group therapists go from child to child to provide support and direction as needed to ensure the children draw the clues that their own bodies give them to signal they are feeling happy (e.g., smile, wide open bright eyes, calm heart).
2. The second drawing is found on page 54 of the same workbook. Children draw their own Body Scan for mad or angry using the large body outline drawn earlier as a template. The child group therapists go from child to child to provide support and direction as needed to ensure the children draw the clues that their own bodies give them to signal they are feeling mad or angry (e.g., tight squeezed eyes, clenched fists, stomping feet and possibly furrowed eyebrows).
3. The third drawing is found on page 1 of the Supplementary Child Workbook. Children draw a picture of themselves practicing Spaghetti Arms and Toes. To facilitate this the lead child group therapist could draw some uncooked spaghetti (e.g., straight, stiff lines) and some cooked spaghetti (e.g., wiggly lines) on the white board (or flip chart) to remind the children to practice Spaghetti Arms and Toes or alternatively, children could draw a picture of themselves lying in bed practicing Spaghetti Arms and Toes (e.g., a stick figure on a bed lying straight).

8.4.6 Part Six of C-Session 1

As seen in Table 8.2, part six of C-Session 1 is Snack Time.

8.4.6.1 Snack Time—General Format for All C-Sessions

Snack Time takes approximately five minutes to complete and follows the same format at each C-Session. After the children complete their craft(s), one of the child group therapists directs them to come to the area set up for snack and distributes the snack. The primary purpose of Snack Time is to facilitate socialization so the child group therapists encourage the children to speak and socialize with each other as well as with the child group therapists. As discussed in Sect. 6.3.3.3, snack consists of healthy and nutritious foods and takes into account allergies, food intolerances, and special dietary requirements. If all group related activities are completed and time permits, the child group therapists could read a short story or play a game (Table 6.3 suggests some stories and games). Alternatively, playing 'I spy with my little eye' is a fun, quick game, that encourages children to take turns, interact with each other and use their voice to speak (or whisper or point for children with selective mutism and/or social anxiety disorder).

8.4.7 Part Seven of C-Session 1

As seen in Table 8.2, part seven of C-Session 1 is wrap up.

8.4.7.1 Wrap up—General Format for All C-Sessions

At each C-Session, wrap up takes less than one minute to complete and follows a structured protocol: In the final few minutes of each C-Session, one child group therapist goes to the parent group room to give a brief (ten seconds or so) summary of what the children learned in the session (e.g., "Today, the children learned____. The children are now ready for you to pick them up"). For this C-Session 1, the child group therapist mentions the name the children chose as their group name. During this time, the other child group therapists assist the children in gathering up their belongings and standing in line to leave the child group room when their parents arrive. Parents come to the child group room to pick up their children and as children leave, the child group therapists encourage the children to say and wave goodbye.

8.5 Step-by-Step Guidelines to Implement C-Session 2

Prior to the start of C-Session 2, the child group therapists decide amongst themselves who leads each component of the session. In C-Session 2, children continue to learn How to Be a Feeling Catcher by doing a Body Scan for nervous or scared and one for shy, review the first relaxation strategy, Spaghetti Arms and Toes, and learn two additional relaxation strategies, Balloon Breathing (a child-friendly way in which to describe diaphragmatic breathing) and Imagery.

Table 8.3 Outline of C-Session 2 (excerpt from Table 6.4)

Session[a]	Child group	
	Minutes	
2	5	Circle Time—reintroduction of children, review of events that might have happened to the children since the last session, and review of topics covered in the previous session
	10	Story Time—Chap. 2 of the children's story[b]—discussion of story
	15	How to Be the Boss of My Body • Balloon Breathing • Imagery How to Be a Feeling Catcher • Body Scans for nervous/scared and shy
	10	Craft Time
	5	Snack Time
	<1	Wrap up

[a]45- to 50-minute session; [b]Children's story section of *Taming Sneaky Fears—Leo the Lion's story of bravery & Inside Leo's den: The workbook* (Benoit & Monga 2018a, b); <: less than

When C-Session 2 is about to start, at least two child and/or parent group therapists greet parents and children in the waiting area and direct the children to the child group room and the parents to the parent group room. The child group therapists are ready to intervene if there are any difficulties with separation. As seen in Table 8.3, there are six parts to C-Session 2.

8.5.1 Part One of C-Session 2

Part one (Circle Time) of C-Session 2 and each subsequent C-Session takes approximately five minutes to complete, begins when all of the children are in the child group room, and includes the following protocol: (1) the child group therapist leading Circle Time distributes the stick-on name tags and re-introduces all the children and therapists; (2) the children are asked if they have anything to share with the group; and (3) the child group therapists take two or three minutes to allow the children to share any information they wish.[7]

The puppets are then distributed and each child chooses a puppet from the container of puppets to hold during the Story Time. Children are asked if they remember Leo the Lion and what happened in the previous session's story. If the children are unable to recall the events of Story Chap. 1, one of the child group therapists provides

---

[7]In subsequent C-Sessions, the child group therapists have additional tasks to complete during Circle Time and these tasks are described in relevant sections of each chapter.

a short synopsis of the story, for example, Leo the Lion is a small lion who feels scared and nervous and is even afraid of his roar but he learned that when he does Spaghetti Arms and Toes he can Be the Boss of his Body.

8.5.2 Part Two of C-Session 2

As seen in Table 8.3, part two of C-Session 2 (Story Time and discussion of story) takes about ten minutes to complete. The child group therapist leading Story Time reads Story Chap. 2 of *Taming Sneaky Fears—Leo the Lion's story of bravery & Inside Leo's den: The workbook* (Benoit & Monga 2018a, b), in a lively and animated tone, while pointing at the illustrations and then discussing the story.

8.5.2.1 Story Discussion

After the story is read, the child group therapist leading the story discussion (three to four minutes in duration) asks if the children liked the story, asks what Leo the Lion learned in the story, and awaits responses such as, Leo the Lion learned that Spaghetti Arms and Toes helps his muscles stay nice and relaxed and Balloon Breathing helps his heart not race and his stomach stop feeling sore; Leo the Lion learned that when he uses Balloon Breathing and Imagery together, he becomes the Boss of his Body and his Brain.

The puppets are returned to the container before moving on to part three.

8.5.3 Part Three of C-Session 2

Part three of C-Session 2 takes about 15 minutes to complete and focuses on two main concepts: (1) How to Be the Boss of My Body by learning how to do Balloon Breathing and Imagery and (2) how to do a Body Scan for nervous or scared and a Body Scan for shy.

8.5.3.1 How to Be the Boss of My Body—Balloon Breathing and Imagery

The child group therapist leading this portion of the session:

1. Asks who practiced using Body Scans and provides verbal praise and stickers to those who did.
2. Asks who practiced Spaghetti Arms and Toes and provides verbal praise and stickers to the children who did.

3. Explains that, just like Leo the Lion did in the story, the children are going to learn two more ways to be the Boss of their Body today.
4. Asks the children what Leo the Lion did in the story to calm his body down when his tummy was sore and his heart was knocking in his chest. If the children are unable to come up with the correct answers, the lead child group therapist reminds them that when Leo used Balloon Breathing, he was able to calm his body down and when he used Balloon Breathing and Imagery together, he was able to calm his body and brain down.

As the child group therapists are about to start teaching the relaxation strategies, they dim the lights (if feasible, ensuring that the room is not too dark). Ideally, children lie down on the floor on a mat as this is more relaxing and children can isolate each muscle group for Spaghetti Arms and Toes and then focus on the movement of their tummy for Balloon Breathing. However, young children can learn each strategy while sitting comfortably in their chairs. The lead child group therapist then reads the Spaghetti Arms and Toes script as described in C-Session 1 (Sect. 8.4.4.4) while the children and the other child group therapists practice Spaghetti Arms and Toes. The child group therapists actively assist the children, as needed, to ensure that the children use the correct techniques.

The lead child group therapist then moves on to Balloon Breathing, which is diaphragmatic or controlled breathing, and follows the script provided in Sect. 8.5.3.2, which is the same script provided in the Parent Manual and similar to the one on p. 60 of the *Taming Sneaky Fears—Leo the Lion's story of bravery & Inside Leo's den: The workbook* (Benoit & Monga 2018a, b). The child group therapists make sure that the children use the proper technique and provide corrective assistance as needed. Although the script suggests that children place one hand on their chest and one hand on their tummy, in the group setting, child group therapists could place a small stuffed animal or puppet on each child's abdomen to help them see the movement of their abdomen. The lead child group therapist could tell the children that they are going to give their puppets (or animals) a slow ride up and down their tummy—if the children complete Balloon Breathing properly the puppet (or animal) on their tummy will rise up when they breathe in and go down then they breathe out. The children practice doing five to six Balloon Breaths in the session before moving on. The lead child group therapist provides verbal praise about how good a job everyone did with the Balloon Breathing and then moves on to explain that just like Leo the Lion did in the story, the children in the group will now learn how to do Imagery together. The lead child group therapist goes on to read in a soothing and calm voice the Imagery script provided in Sect. 8.5.3.3 (which is the same script found in the Parent Manual and similar to the one on p. 61 of the *Taming Sneaky Fears—Leo the Lion's story of bravery & Inside Leo's den: The workbook* (Benoit & Monga 2018a, b).

8.5.3.2 Balloon Breathing Script

Put one of your hands on your tummy, just above your belly button, and the other hand on your chest. Make sure the hand on your chest doesn't move at all and your shoulders are relaxed when you do Balloon Breathing. The hand on your tummy will move up and down as the air goes in and out of your tummy when you do Balloon Breathing. *If a small stuffed animal (or puppet) is being used then these are placed on the child's abdomen and the therapist explains that the stuffed animal (or puppet) is going to go for a slow ride up and down on the child's tummy.* Take a really slow breath in through your nose. Pretend your tummy is a balloon and when you breathe in, let the air go down to your tummy, and let your tummy fill up with air just like a big balloon. Now hold the air in your tummy balloon and count to five slowly—one, two, three, four, five. Now slowly let the air out from your tummy-balloon and push it out of your mouth like you're blowing out a birthday candle. Let's hear you blowing those candles out. Now do that again. Relax your shoulders. Take a breath in through your nose and let the air go down to your tummy so that your tummy gets big like a balloon and now count to five slowly—one, two, three, four, five. Now slowly breathe out and push the air out through your mouth like you're blowing out a birthday candle. Let's do this five more times, really slowly (*the lead child group therapist repeats the script as the children continue to do five more Balloon Breaths*). Make sure you relax your shoulders. Make sure your shoulders and chest don't move at all and that only your belly moves up and down when you do the Balloon Breathing.

8.5.3.3 Script for Imagery

Close your eyes and pretend or imagine that you're lying on a beach on a beautiful sunny day. Imagine the bright yellow sun shining. You see fluffy white clouds in the blue sky. The sun is warm and feels so good on your skin. You hear the soft whisper of a gentle breeze. The air smells fresh and clean. The white sand is warm and soft and feels really, really good. You can hear the waves coming in and going out. The sound of the waves makes you feel safe, calm, and relaxed. You think about building a sand castle, but right now it feels so good to just lie here on the soft, warm sand. You let the bright sun shine on you. You hear the waves come in and go out. You feel safe, warm, comfortable, and so relaxed. Just imagine for a few more minutes the fluffy white clouds in the blue sky as they float by above you, the soft sound of the waves, the feel of the warm sun on your skin, and the smell of the salty, clean sea air. Now slowly open our eyes.

8.5.3.4 How to Be a Feeling Catcher and Use a Body Scan

After completing the relaxation strategies, the child group therapist leading the discussion uses a large laminated picture of genderless child body outline or draws a large child body outline on the white board (or flip chart) for this portion of the session. Using the steps described in Sect. 8.4.4.2, the lead child group therapist completes a Body Scan for nervous or scared and a Body Scan for shy. This is done by asking the children to think about how each body part, starting from their head and moving down to their toes, looks and feels like when they are feeling nervous or scared (and later when they feel shy). As done in the previous session, the child group therapist leading this section could ask the children to make a scared or nervous (and later a shy) face to begin the discussion. The lead child group therapist again draws the suggestions provided by the children and child group therapists on the large body outline.

For C-Session 2, the completed Body Scan for nervous or scared could show a heart beating fast, hard and stiff muscles like uncooked spaghetti (straight lines in the extremities), and sore stomach (butterflies could be drawn in the stomach area), while the Body Scan for shy could show downcast eyes, red cheeks, squeezed throat or voice that is stuck and will not come out (color in the throat area), and muscles stiff and hard like uncooked spaghetti (straight lines in the arms and legs).

The lead child group therapist reminds the children that when they pay attention to the clues their body gives them by doing a Body Scan, they can figure out and 'catch' if they are feeling happy, mad or angry, nervous or scared, shy, sad, or any other feeling. The lead child group therapist emphasizes the importance of practicing Body Scans every day so that the children become better Feeling Catchers, just like Leo the Lion!

8.5.4 Part Four of C-Session 2

As seen in Table 8.3, part four of C-Session 2 is Craft Time, follows the format outlined in Sect. 8.4.5.1, and takes about ten minutes to complete.

8.5.4.1 Specific Craft for C-Session 2

One of the child group therapists leads the craft activity by explaining what is required and demonstrating what to draw on the white board (or flip chart) as needed. The other child group therapists distribute the required workbooks, ensure that the children are on the correct page, and go from child to child to provide the children with the support and direction they require for each drawing. Craft Time for C-Session 2 has three drawings:

1. The first drawing is on page 57 of the workbook section of *Taming Sneaky Fears—Leo the Lion's story of bravery & Inside Leo's Den: The workbook* (Benoit & Monga 2018a, b).[8] Children draw their own Body Scan for nervous or

---

[8]The workbook section of *Taming Sneaky Fears—Leo the Lion's story of bravery & Inside Leo's den: The workbook* (Benoit & Monga 2018a, b) contains a number of other drawings that children could do; however, due to time constraints of the group sessions, these drawings are not done in the

scared using the large body outline drawn earlier as a template. The child group therapists go from child to child to provide support and direction as needed to ensure the children draw the clues that their own bodies give them to signal they are feeling nervous or scared.

2. The second drawing is on page 58 of the workbook section of *Taming Sneaky Fears—Leo the Lion's story of bravery & Inside Leo's Den: The workbook* (Benoit & Monga 2018a, b). Children draw their own Body Scan for shy using the large body outline drawn earlier as a template. The child group therapists go from child to child to provide support and direction as needed to ensure the children draw the clues that their own bodies give them to signal they are feeling shy.

3. The third craft is on page 2 of the Supplementary Child Workbook. The children draw a picture of themselves practicing Balloon Breathing. To facilitate this, the lead child group therapist could draw on the white board (or flip chart) a child (e.g., a stick figure) with balloons (lines with round circles at the top) around to remind the children that they are practicing Balloon Breathing or the child lying in bed practicing Balloon Breathing.

4. If time permits, the children could draw a picture of the safe and calm place they imagine when they are doing Imagery, using the space provided on page 62 of the workbook section of *Taming Sneaky Fears—Leo the Lion's story of bravery & Inside Leo's Den: The workbook* (Benoit & Monga 2018a, b). If this craft is completed within the group session, the child group therapists ensure that the children draw a calm place, not a place that is happy or exciting and ensure the children incorporate all five senses in their drawing (i.e., what they see, hear, smell, taste, and touch or feel on their skin).

8.5.5 Part Five of C-Session 2

Part five of C-Session 2 is Snack Time and follows the protocol outlined in Sect. 8.4.6.1.

8.5.6 Part Six of C-Session 2

Part six of Child-Session 2 is wrap up and follows the protocol outlined in Sect. 8.4.7.1.

---

group (during the parent group sessions and at the final Session 8 (graduation), parents are informed that there are additional drawings that they could encourage their children to do to help the children further integrate what they have learned during the group program).

Table 8.4 Outline of C-Session 5 (excerpt from Table 6.4)

Session[a]	Child group	
	Minutes	
5	*Child group therapists meet with each child's parent(s) for five minutes **at the end of Session 4** and (as needed) **immediately prior to the beginning of Session 5** to provide and receive feedback on the child's progress*	
	5–10	Circle Time—review of events that might have happened to the children since the last session, relaxation strategies, and concepts from C-Sessions 3 and 4 (Tricks, Stop sign, and Trick Stoppers)
	10	Story Time—Chap. 5 of the children's story[b] and discussion of story
	15	How to Be a Feeling Catcher • Feeling Thermometer
	10	Craft Time
	5	Snack Time
	<1	Wrap up

[a]45- to 50-minute session; [b]Children's story section of *Taming Sneaky Fears—Leo the Lion's story of bravery & Inside Leo's den: The workbook* (Benoit & Monga, 2018a, b); <: less than

8.6 Step-by-Step Guidelines to Implement C-Session 5

C-Session 5 is the final C-Session that makes up the child component of feeling recognition and management in the Taming Sneaky Fears program. The key concept for children to learn in C-Session 5 is how to use the Feeling Thermometer to rate feeling intensity. By C-Session 5, most children have a good understanding of feeling recognition (i.e., they know How to Be a Feeling Catcher and do Body Scans) and are proficient in using the relaxation strategies to Be the Boss of their Body, providing they and their parents have practiced the various relaxations strategies at home as instructed. As with other C-Sessions, prior to the start of C-Session 5, the child group therapists decide their respective roles in the session. At the appropriate start time, at least two child and/or parent group therapists go to the waiting room and direct the parents and children to the parent and child group rooms. As seen in Table 8.4, there are six parts to C-Session 5.

8.6.1 Part One of C-Session 5

Part one of C-Session 5 (Circle Time), which takes 5–10 minutes to complete, begins when all the children are in the child group room. Part one follows the protocol used to begin each C-Session as outlined in Sect. 8.5.1, which includes distribution of name tags, inviting the children to share things about their time since the last session for a minute or two, asking the children if they practiced their relaxation strategies and providing verbal praise and/or stickers to those who practiced, and practicing Spaghetti Arms and Toes and Balloon Breathing, Balloon Breathing, and Imagery for a few minutes.

In addition, for the next five to seven minutes, the child group therapist taking the lead for Circle Time:

1. Asks the children if they remember Sneaky Fears and how sneaky Sneaky Fears can be. Most children are quite enamored by Sneaky Fears and can get quite excited talking about the characters.
2. Reminds the children that in order to tame Sneaky Fears they have to learn How to Be the Boss of their Brain, just like Leo the Lion did in the story.
3. Reviews How to Be a Trick Catcher in order to catch the Tricks that Sneaky Fears play by reminding the children that when they feel nervous or scared or some other yucky feeling, it usually means that Sneaky Fears are playing Tricks on their brain, and when they become Trick Catchers and 'catch' (or recognize) the Tricks that Sneaky Fears play, they become the Boss of their Brain.
4. Asks the children to name the three Tricks that Sneaky Fears play (i.e., Not Telling the Truth, Exaggerating, and Only Showing the Bad Things) and the three Trick Stoppers (i.e., Ignore Sneaky Fears, Think Brave Thoughts, and Talk to an Adult). The lead child group therapist encourages the children to call out the various Tricks and Trick Stoppers, making sure to write these down on the white board (or flip chart).

The puppets are then distributed and each child chooses a puppet from the container of puppets to hold during the Story Time.

8.6.2 Part Two of C-Session 5

As seen in Table 8.4, part two of C-Session 2 (Story Time and discussion of story) takes about ten minutes to complete. The child group therapist leading Story Time reads Story Chap. 5 of *Taming Sneaky Fears—Leo the Lion's story of bravery & Inside Leo's den: The workbook* (Benoit & Monga 2018a, b), in a lively and animated tone, while pointing at the illustrations and then discussing the story.

8.6.2.1 Story Discussion

After the story has been read, the child group therapist leading the story discussion (three to four minutes in duration) asks if the children like the story and what happened to Leo the Lion in the story. The lead child group therapist supports the children to come up with (and/or provides) responses such as, Leo the Lion went to Ellie the

Elephant's house for a play date and when he saw Ellie's brother Elliot having his temperature taken with a fever thermometer, Leo and Ellie figured out that they could use a Feeling Thermometer to gauge the intensity of their feelings, and they figure out when they are at a 5 or more on their Feeling Thermometer, they are way too upset to think clearly and they have to use Spaghetti Arms and Toes, Balloon Breathing, or Imagery to get their Feeling Thermometer down to a 1 or a 2 and calm their body down so they can think clearly. Before moving on to part three, the puppets are returned to the container.

8.6.3   Part Three of C-Session 5

As seen in Table 8.4, part three of C-Session 5 (How to Be a Feeling Catcher) takes about 15 minutes to complete and consists of showing the children how and why to use the Feeling Thermometer (Fig. 8 in the Parent Manual). The child group therapist leading this portion of the session uses a large, laminated illustration of the Feeling Thermometer or draws one on the white board (or flip chart). If the lead child group therapist draws a Feeling Thermometer, three boxes are also drawn beside the Feeling Thermometer, one near the bottom of the Feeling Thermometer, one near the middle of the Feeling Thermometer and one near the top of the Feeling Thermometer (much like the illustration on page 77 in the workbook section of *Taming Sneaky Fears—Leo the Lion's story of bravery & Inside Leo's den: The workbook* (Benoit & Monga 2018a, b). The lead child group therapist:

1. Asks if the children can remember how Ellie the Elephant felt when her cousin said "Boo," and reminds the children that Ellie felt a 1 or 2 on the Feeling Thermometer, i.e., just a little scared.
2. Asks and encourages the children to come up with their own examples of situations when they felt a 1 or a 2 on the Feeling Thermometer for nervous or scared, and writes these down (or draws something to represent these situations) close to the bottom (or in the bottom box) of the large Feeling Thermometer.
3. Asks and encourages the children to come up with their own examples of situations when they felt a 5 or a 6 on the Feeling Thermometer for nervous or scared, and writes these down (or draws something to represent these situations) close to the middle (or in the middle box) of the large Feeling Thermometer.
4. Asks and encourages the children to come up with their own examples of situations when they felt a 9 or a 10 on the Feeling Thermometer for nervous or scared, and writes these down (or draws something to represent these situations) close to the top (or in the top box) of the large Feeling Thermometer.
5. Provides (along with the other child group therapists) child-friendly examples of situations as needed if the children are having a difficult time coming up with appropriate examples, again with the goal of using examples that are pertinent to the symptoms of anxiety experienced by the children attending the group.

6. Completes a second Feeling Thermometer for feeling shy, following the afore-mentioned steps 2–5 and encouraging the children to provide situations when they felt a little shy, shy at a 5 or 6, and shy at a 9 or 10 (and draws or write these situations) at the corresponding points of the large Feeling Thermometer.
7. Emphasizes that for each child, different situations may cause different intensities of nervous or scared and shy feelings.
8. Reviews what Leo the Lion said about how they cannot think clearly when they are at a 5 or higher on the Feeling Thermometer and that means they need to use their relaxation strategies to bring down the Feeling Thermometer to a 1 or 2.
9. Explains that when their Feeling Thermometer is higher than a 5 on the Feeling Thermometer for nervous or scared, or the Feeling Thermometer for shy, or the Feeling Thermometer for any other yucky feeling like angry or mad or sad, that means Sneaky Fears are playing Tricks on their brain.
10. Emphasizes that when their Feeling Thermometer is at a 5 or higher that means they need to do Spaghetti Arms and Toes, Balloon Breathing, and Imagery to calm their body down so that they become the Boss of their Body, just like Leo the Lion did in the story.
11. Reminds the children that only when their body is calm, can they think clearly and can they be a Trick Catcher to catch the Tricks that Sneaky Fears are playing, use the Stop sign, and use the Trick Stoppers (Ignore Sneaky Fears, Think Brave Thoughts, and Talk to an Adult).

8.6.4 Part Four of C-Session 5

As seen in Table 8.4, part four of C-Session 5 is Craft Time, follows the format outlined in Sect. 8.4.5.1, and takes about ten minutes to complete.

8.6.4.1 Specific Craft for C-Session 5

One of the child group therapists leads the craft activity by explaining what is required and demonstrating what to draw on the white board (or flip chart) as needed. The other child group therapists distribute the two workbooks and ensure the children are on the correct page when completing each drawing. The lead child group therapist ensures that the large Feeling Thermometers created during the session are visible to the children during the completion of the crafts. The child group therapists also provide individual support and ideas for situations that represent the different intensities on the Feeling Thermometer for nervous or scared and later on with the second craft, ideas for situations that represent the different intensities on the Feeling Thermometer for shy. Craft Time for C-Session 5 has two drawings:

1. The first drawing is on page 77 of the workbook section of *Taming Sneaky Fears—Leo the Lion's story of bravery & Inside Leo's den: The workbook* (Benoit & Monga 2018a, b). Children draw a situation that makes them feel a 1 or 2 on their Feeling Thermometer for nervous or scared in the bottom box, a situation that makes them feel a 5 or 6 on their Feeling Thermometer for nervous or scared in the middle box, and a situation that makes them feel a 9 or 10 on their Feeling Thermometer for nervous or scared in the top box.

2. The second drawing is on page 4 of the Supplementary Child Workbook. Children follow the same instructions provided for their first craft, but this time they draw situations that make them feel a 1 or 2 (in the bottom box), then a 5 or 6 (in the middle box), then a 9 or 10 (in the top box) on their Feeling Thermometer for shy.

8.6.5 Part Five of C-Session 5

Part five of C-Session 5 is Snack Time and follows the protocol outlined in Sect. 8.4.6.1.

8.6.6 Part Six of C-Session 5

Part six of C-Session 5 is wrap up and follows the protocol outlined in Sect. 8.4.7.1.

References

Benoit, D., & Monga, S. (2018a). *Apprivoiser les Peurs-pas-fines—L'histoire de bravoure de Léo le lionceau & Dans la tanière de Léo: Le cahier de travail*. Victoria, British Columbia: FriesenPress.

Benoit, D., & Monga, S. (2018b). *Taming sneaky fears—Leo the Lion's story of bravery & Inside Leo's den: The workbook*. Victoria, British Columbia: FriesenPress.

Koeppen, A. S. (1974). Relaxation training for children. *Elementary School Guidance & Counseling, 9,* 14–21.

Manassis, K. (2008). *Keys to parenting your anxious child* (2nd ed.). Hauppauge, NY: Barron's Educational Series.

Chapter 9
The Taming Sneaky Fears Program: How to Be a Trick Catcher and the Boss of My Brain

9.1 Overview and Rationale

Young children need help to understand the complex and abstract concept of cognitive distortions. As described in Sect. 6.1.1.1, in the Taming Sneaky Fears program, anxiety is externalized as Sneaky Fears and the concept of cognitive distortions is rendered more concrete by referring to the Tricks that Sneaky Fears play by sneaking untrue, negative thoughts in children's brain and tricking them into believing these thoughts are true. The various cognitive distortions are further simplified into three overarching Tricks: Not Telling the Truth, Exaggerating, and Only Showing the Bad Things. Through the children's story and companion workbook, *Taming Sneaky Fears—Leo the Lion's story of bravery & Inside Leo's den: The Workbook* (Benoit & Monga, 2018a, b), children hear how Leo the Lion learns to be brave and tame his Sneaky Fears by using Trick Stoppers (or cognitive coping strategies, including Ignore Sneaky Fears, Think Brave Thoughts, and Talk to an Adult). The concept of cognitive distortions (the Tricks that Sneaky Fears play) and cognitive coping strategies (the Trick Stoppers and an additional strategy discussed in group, the Stop sign) are introduced to the parents in one session (P-Session 2) and to the children in two sessions (C-Sessions 3 and 4).

9.2 Step-by-Step Guidelines to Implement P-Session 2

Prior to the start of P-Session 2, the parent group therapists determine which therapists are in charge of which specific parts of P-Session 2 and ensure that all the materials needed (as listed in Table 6.3) are available in the parent group room.

© Springer Nature Switzerland AG 2018
S. Monga and D. Benoit, *Assessing and Treating Anxiety Disorders in Young Children*, https://doi.org/10.1007/978-3-030-04939-3_9

Table 9.1 Outline of P-Session 2 (excerpt from Table 6.4)

Session[a]	Parent group	
	Minutes	
2	5	Parents volunteer examples of brave moments and effective praise
	5	Review of other tasks

	30-40	How to be a Trick Catcher and catch the Tricks that Sneaky Fears play
		 • Not Telling the Truth
		 • Exaggerating
		 • Only Showing the Bad Things
		 How to Be the Boss of My Brain
		 • Use the Stop sign
		 • Use the Trick Stoppers
		   – Ignore Sneaky Fears
		   – Think Brave Thoughts
		   – Talk to an Adult

	<1	Wrap up

[a]45- to 50-minute session; children and parent groups run concurrently, but in separate rooms; <: less than

As P-Session 2 is about to start, at least two child and/or parent group therapists go to the waiting area to greet all parents and children and bring them to their respective room.[1]

As the parents enter the parent group room, one of the parent group therapists welcomes them and invites them to take their name tag from the table and put it on as they make themselves comfortable. If parents are in charge of bringing the snack for the child group session, the lead parent group therapist thanks the parent who brought the snack and reminds the parents of which parent is in charge of bringing the children's snack for the next session.

9.2.1 Part One of P-Session 2

As seen in Table 9.1, P-Session 2 in the Taming Sneaky Fears program is divided into four parts. Part one of P-Session 2 (brave moments and effective praise) takes approximately five minutes to complete and follows the protocol outlined in Sect. 8.3.2, i.e., the parent group therapist leading this part of P-Session 2 asks two or three parents to volunteer examples of brave moments they noticed in their children since the previous session and how they provided effective praise. The lead parent group therapist encourages parent engagement by:

---

[1]If parents are in charge of bringing the snacks for the child group sessions, it is typically at that moment that the parent who brings the snack gives it to one of the child group therapists.

1. Inviting supportive comments from other parents on what the parents volunteering examples did well when providing effective praise and what they could have done differently to provide even more effective praise.
2. Asking parents to review the three main characteristics of effective praise (i.e., start praise with a '*You*' statement, focus on *the specific behavior* displayed by the child, provide praise *as soon as possible* after the display of the brave behavior).
3. Asking parents to explain the rationale for identifying brave moments and providing effective praise (i.e., the more one pays attention to a behavior, the more likely the behavior is to be repeated).

Throughout this part, the parent group therapists actively provide constructive feedback to the parents who volunteer examples and comments. The parent group therapists remind the parents that focusing on brave moments and providing effective praise are tasks to do throughout the program (and ideally, would continue even after the Taming Sneaky Fears program is completed).

9.2.2 Part Two of P-Session 2

Part two of P-Session 2 (review of other tasks) takes approximately five minutes to complete. One parent group therapist takes the lead for this part and completes the following tasks:

1. Asks the parents to volunteer how they encouraged their children to practice doing Body Scans and Spaghetti Arms and Toes.
2. Promotes parent engagement by inviting comments on what the parents volunteering examples did well when they encouraged their children to practice doing Body Scans (and/or charades) and Spaghetti Arms and Toes, and what they could do if their children show resistance to doing Body Scans (and/or charades) and practicing Spaghetti Arms and Toes.
3. Reminds the parents that today in the children's group, the children are learning to do a Body Scan for nervous or scared, a Body Scan for shy, Balloon Breathing, and Imagery.
4. Encourages the parents to continue doing Body Scans (and/or charades) and practice all relaxation strategies with their children using the practice charts provided in the Parent Manual[2] (Fig. 14 for Spaghetti Arms and Toes, Fig. 15 for Balloon Breathing, and Fig. 16 for Balloon Breathing and Imagery together).

9.2.3 Part Three of P-Session 2

Part three of P-Session 2 is content heavy and the parent group therapists mention this to the parents and pace themselves to ensure they can cover all the materials

---

[2]The Parent Manual is provided as part of the Supplementary Materials in Chap. 6.

for P-Session 2. Part three takes 30–40 minutes to complete. To begin part three of P-Session 2, the parent group therapist leading this portion:

1. Shows the children's two workbooks, i.e., the workbook section of *Taming Sneaky Fears—Leo the Lion's story of bravery & Inside Leo's den: The workbook* (Benoit & Monga, 2018a, b) and the Supplementary Child Workbook,[3] to the parents and points out the drawings the children are doing during today's session: a drawing that shows How to Be a Feeling Catcher by doing a Body Scan for nervous or scared and a Body Scan for shy, and a drawing of How to Be the Boss of My Body by doing Balloon Breathing. If time allows, the children might be able to draw a picture of their safe and calm place when they do Imagery.
2. Reminds the parents that they do not have the children's workbooks in their possession, as these are kept with the child group therapists until Session 8 ('graduation') when the children's workbooks are given to the children to take home; mentions to the parents that the workbook section of the *Taming Sneaky Fears—Leo the Lion's story of bravery & Inside Leo's den: The workbook* (Benoit & Monga, 2018a, b) contains more activities the children could do than time allows in the group sessions, so at the end of the group program, parents could complete these additional activities with the children to help them further integrate the concepts they have learned during the group sessions.
3. Mentions that the parents can use Figs. 10–16 from their Parent Manual until the next session to get their children to practice being Feeling Catchers, doing Body Scans, and using the three relaxation strategies (Spaghetti Arms and Toes, Balloon Breathing, and Imagery).
4. Emphasizes the importance for parents to ensure that their children master the concepts of being Feeling Catchers and doing Body Scans, and use the correct techniques when doing Spaghetti Arms and Toes, Balloon Breathing, and Imagery (and reiterates the need for children to practice each relaxation strategy for at least five minutes, every day, when they are relaxed and do not need the relaxation strategy); without mastering these concepts and skills, the children might struggle with the next components of the Taming Sneaky Fears program.
5. Mentions that the children practice each relaxation strategy under the child group therapist's supervision at the beginning of each session, starting with today's Session 2 and receive stickers for having practiced at home.
6. Mentions that after they master the relaxation strategies, children are likely to develop a preference for one or two relaxation strategies that they find work(s) best for them (for now, we ask that parents expose their children to all three relaxation strategies until they are mastered).
7. Uses the laminated copy of Fig. 6.2 (or Fig. 3 from the Parent Manual) illustrating the overlap between traditional CBT and the Taming Sneaky Fears program to remind the parents that at the last session, the focus was on the 'Feeling' component of the cognitive triangle while during today's parent session the focus

---

[3]The Supplementary Child Workbook is provided as part of the Supplementary Materials in Chap. 6.

is on the 'Thought' component of the cognitive triangle; so in today's session, parents learn the following concepts:

a. Sneaky Fears (i.e., *externalize* anxiety).
b. The Tricks that Sneaky Fears play (cognitive distortions).
c. How to Be a Trick Catcher and catch the Tricks that Sneaky Fears play (the lead parent group therapist indicates that the children learn about Sneaky Fears, the Tricks that Sneaky Fears play, and How to Be a Trick Catcher at their next two sessions, so the lead parent group therapist asks parents to refrain from using the terms Sneaky Fears, the Tricks that Sneaky Fears play, and How to Be a Trick Catcher until these concepts are introduced in the child sessions).
d. How to Be the Boss of My Brain by using the Stop sign and the Trick Stoppers; the lead parent group therapist indicates that the children learn about these concepts in the next two sessions and asks parents to refrain from using the terms How to Be the Boss of My Brain by using the Stop sign and the Trick Stoppers until the terminology is introduced in the child sessions.
e. Uses the laminated copy of the What to Do to Help list (Fig. 4 of the Parent Manual) to point out that the foci of today's session are on items 6 and 7 of that list.

9.2.3.1   How to Be a Trick Catcher

The parent group therapist leading this portion:

1. Asks the parents to go to Session 2 in their Parent Manual (and points to the page number where Session 2 begins).
2. Encourages the parents to follow along as the parent group therapist covers the materials from Session 2 in the Parent Manual.
3. Draws (on a dry-erase board or flip chart) a cognitive triangle with the words 'Thought,' 'Feeling,' and 'Behavior' written at each point/angle of the triangle and a separate rectangle with the word 'Situation' in it near the top left of the triangle (as in Fig. 6.1 or Fig. 2 of the Parent Manual; the lead parent therapist could draw the cognitive triangle prior to the beginning of the P-Session 2), and

    a. Describes the following 'Situation:' "You walk into a restaurant and you see two of your friends sitting at a table and carrying a conversation. As they lift their heads up and see you, they look at each other and burst out laughing" (the parent group therapist writes a summary of this situation next to the 'Situation' rectangle).
    b. Asks the parents what first thought would come to mind in this situation.
    c. Lets the parents provide examples of various thoughts and when a parent provides an example that is along the lines of, 'they're laughing at me,' the lead parent group therapist writes down this response next to the 'Thought' point/angle of the cognitive triangle, using a marker (the ink color does not

matter, what matters is that the same color is used to write down the corresponding feeling and behavior generated by that one thought).

d. Asks the parents something like, "If the thought that comes to mind when 'you walk into the restaurant and see your two friends burst out laughing as soon as they see you' was 'they're laughing at me,' how would that make you feel?"

e. Lets the parents provide examples of feelings that such a thought would generate and writes down one of those feelings (typically a negative feeling, such as embarrassed, shy, upset).

f. Writes down a few relevant parents' responses next to the Feeling point/angle of the triangle, in the same color as the thought that generated that feeling.

g. Asks the parents how intense that feeling would be on the Feeling Thermome-ter (if the thought that came to mind when they walked into the restaurant and saw two friends burst out laughing as soon as they saw them was 'they're laughing at me'); the parents are likely to say a 7 or above.

h. Then asks the parents what they would do if they felt that negative emotion at a 7 or more on the Feeling Thermometer when the thought that came to mind when they walked into the restaurant and saw two friends burst out laughing as soon as they saw them was 'they're laughing at me.'

i. Lets the parents provide examples of responses, chooses a response that relates to 'avoidance' (e.g., turn around and walk out of the restaurant; in other words, avoid the situation), points out that avoidance is a typical response of anxious children who face anxiety-provoking situations, and writes down the response next to 'Behavior' point/angle of the triangle, using the same color of marker in which the 'Thought' and 'Feeling' had been written.

j. Turns to the cognitive triangle the group has just completed and points out that when a situation has happened, it cannot be changed; one does not have control over a situation that has already happened. What one has control over is what one makes of the situation (i.e., the thought that one generates in a given situation). In turn, that thought affects how one feels (and how intensely one feels the emotion) and what one does (behavior); so thoughts, feelings, and behaviors are all inter-related.

k. Focuses on the 'Thought' component of the cognitive triangle and explains (while writing down next to the word 'Thought') that thoughts can be:
    i. Accurate or inaccurate (inaccurate thoughts are cognitive distortions).
    ii. Helpful or unhelpful (a thought is unhelpful if it generates a negative feeling).

l. Mentions that children with anxiety disorders typically generate automatic, inaccurate, and unhelpful thoughts in various situations (e.g., 'everybody is going to laugh at me,' 'my voice sounds weird,' 'mommy is going to forget me places,' 'something bad is going to happen if mommy leaves').

m. Asks the parents to generate a thought that would be more accurate and more helpful for the same situation ('you walk into the restaurant and see your two friends burst out laughing as soon as they see you') and writes down the parents' responses, using a different color marker; parents will likely come up with something like 'they just told a funny joke.'

n. Asks the parents what they would feel if 'they just told a funny joke' was the thought that came to mind in the same situation; parents are likely to say something like 'I would feel ok, good.'

o. Points out that the thought, 'they just told a funny joke' is a helpful thought because it generates a positive or neutral feeling (and probably a feeling that is lower than a 5 on the Feeling Thermometer); it would be difficult to determine whether the thought is more accurate unless one would approach the friends and check with them.

p. Asks the parents what they would do if the thought that came to mind was 'they just told a joke' and that thought made them feel 'ok, good' (parents are likely to say something along the lines of "approach the friends" and the parent group therapist writes down this answer next to the 'Behavior' point/angle of the cognitive triangle, using the second color that was used with the second thought and feeling).

q. Emphasizes that in the two scenarios above, the situation is the same; the difference is what one makes of the situation (thought) and in turn, what one makes of the situation affects how one feels (feeling) and what one does (behavior).

r. Explains that, as described in the Parent Manual (and points out the page in the Parent Manual where this information is found), in the Taming Sneaky Fears program, we tackle the concept of inaccurate and unhelpful thoughts (or cognitive distortions) by introducing the Tricks that Sneaky Fears play (the parent group therapist reminds parents briefly that in a previous session, we talked about *externalizing* anxiety and making it concrete by calling it Sneaky Fears and using two jackal characters in the story and two jackal-like puppets in the group to make Sneaky Fears come to life).

s. Describes that in the children's story that is read to the children in the group, *Taming Sneaky Fears—Leo the Lion's story of bravery & Inside Leo's den: The workbook* (Benoit & Monga, 2018a, b), Sneaky Fears are two annoying and bothersome jackal characters that keep putting negative, inaccurate, and unhelpful thoughts (cognitive distortions) in Leo the Lion's brain.

t. Mentions that, as described in the Parent Manual (and points to the page where this information is located), all young anxious children's own Sneaky Fears *sneak* untrue and scary (inaccurate and unhelpful) thoughts in their brain (e.g., 'people will laugh at me if I speak,' 'there are monsters under my bed,' 'something bad is going to happen to mommy when I'm at school,' etc.).

u. Mentions that starting at their next group session, the children will be introduced to Sneaky Fears and will learn that these untrue and scary (or inaccurate and unhelpful) thoughts are Tricks (or cognitive distortions) that Sneaky Fears play. The children will also learn that these Tricks that Sneaky Fears play make Leo the Lion and his friend, Ellie the Elephant, feel a negative emotion (e.g., shy, scared or nervous, etc.), which, in turn, affects their behavior negatively (e.g., Leo avoids talking to his teacher and peers, Ellie avoids trying to do new things, both Leo and Ellie avoid facing their fears).

  v. Mentions that in the group, the children will learn that their own Sneaky Fears try to play Tricks on their brain and so they need to learn to be Trick Catchers to figure out and 'catch' the Tricks that their own Sneaky Fears are playing on their brain; learning how to 'catch' the Tricks that Sneaky Fears play is an important step before children can learn to tame their Sneaky Fears.

  w. Mentions that the children also learn that all the Sneaky Fears in the world know only three Tricks: Not Telling the Truth, Exaggerating, and Only Showing the Bad Things.

  x. Directs the parents to the two Scripts for Learning How to Be a Trick Catcher (i.e., one script to be used before Session 5 and one script to be used after Session 5; does not read the scripts, only mentions that the parents could use them if they wish and that the difference between the two scripts pertains to the fact that in Session 5, the children learn about the Feeling Thermometer, so there is a mention of the Feeling Thermometer in the After Session 5 script).

9.2.3.2   How to Be the Boss of My Brain

The parent group therapist leading this portion:

1. Asks the parent to go to Fig. 19 in the Parent Manual (and points out the page number where this information is located) while using Fig. 3 of the Parent Manual to highlight that after the children learn How to Be a Trick Catcher and catch the Tricks that Sneaky Fears play, they find out How to Be the Boss of My Brain (and not let Sneaky Fears be the boss of their brain).

2. Directs the parents' attention to Fig. 20 of the Parent Manual, which summarizes How to Be the Boss of My Body and highlights How to Be the Boss of My Brain, by using the Stop sign and the Trick Stoppers, Ignore Sneaky Fears, Think Brave Thoughts, and Talk to an Adult.

3. Spends three or four minutes summarizing the script for the Stop sign (and indicates to the parents where they can find the script in their Parent Manual) by saying that children learn that when they make their brain think of all the elements of a Stop sign (shape, color, letters, color of letters), their brain is so busy thinking about all these things that their brain has no time to think about worries or the scary and untrue thoughts that Sneaky Fears are trying to sneak into their brain; this means that the children become the Boss of their Brain and do not let Sneaky Fears be the boss of their brain (this strategy is similar to the Trick Stopper, Ignore Sneaky Fears, and essentially uses a form of 'distraction') as it helps children ignore Sneaky Fears.

4. Points out to the parents that they could use this script when discussing the Stop sign with their children (or could ask their children how and when to use the Stop sign; this way, parents can determine if their children understand the concept).

5. Directs the parents' attention to the script for How to Be the Boss of My Brain (and points out where parents can find the script in their Parent Manual); the parent group therapist does not read the entire script, but only emphasizes that when children 'catch' Sneaky Fears playing Tricks on their brain (a sure sign that Sneaky Fears are playing their Tricks is when one feels a negative emotion at a 5 or more on the Feeling Thermometer), children can decide to not let Sneaky Fears be the boss of their brain, i.e., children can:

   a. Decide to make their brain think of the Stop sign (instead of the scary and untrue thoughts that Sneaky Fears are trying to sneak into their brain).
   b. Then make their brain do Imagery and think of their safe and calm place (and not the scary and untrue thoughts that Sneaky Fears are trying to sneak into their brain).
   c. Do relaxation strategies to get their body to calm down so their brain can think more clearly.
   d. Use the Trick Stoppers to tame their Sneaky Fears (the lead parent group therapist directs the parents' attention to the section on the Trick Stoppers (and points out where the parents can find the information in their Parent Manual):
       i.   Ignore Sneaky Fears.
       ii. Think Brave Thoughts.
       iii. Talk to an Adult.

6. Reviews the Parent Session 2 Tasks (and points out where parents can find this information in their Parent Manual).

9.2.4 Part Four of P-Session 2

Part four of P-Session 2 (wrap up) takes 30–60 seconds to complete and follows the protocol outlined in Sect. 8.3.4.

9.3 Step-by-Step Guidelines to Implement C-Session 3

The first key concept the children learn in C-Session 3 is that their anxiety symptoms come, in large part, from scary and untrue thoughts (cognitive distortions) that their brain automatically thinks about in some anxiety-provoking situations. To help young children understand this abstract concept, anxiety is *externalized* as Sneaky Fears, these annoying twin jackals that keep bothering the main story character, Leo the Lion, by putting scary and untrue thoughts in Leo's brain. To further externalize anxiety, the Sneaky Fears puppets 'come alive' through the story as one of the child group therapists brings these puppets out at the appropriate times during the story telling and reads the words that Sneaky Fears say in a snarling and somewhat scary

Table 9.2 Outline of C-Session 3 (excerpt from Table 6.4)

Session[a]	Child group	
	Minutes	
3	5–10	Circle Time—review of events that might have happened to the children since the last session, topics covered in the previous session, and relaxation strategies
	10	Story Time—Chap. 3 of children's story[b] meet Sneaky Fears and discussion of story

	15	How to be a Trick Catcher
		• Trick #1: Not Telling the Truth
		How to Be the Boss of My Brain:
		• Use the Stop sign
		• Use the Trick Stoppers
		  – Ignore Sneaky Fears
		  – Think Brave Thoughts

	10	Craft Time
	5	Snack Time
	<1	Wrap up

[a]45- to 50-minute session; [b]Children's story section of *Taming Sneaky Fears—Leo the Lion's story of bravery & Inside Leo's den: The workbook* (Benoit & Monga, 2018a, b); <: less than

voice. In the group, children learn that when their own Sneaky Fears put scary and untrue thoughts in their own brain, they feel really nervous, scared, or shy. And when they feel that nervous, scared, or shy, they cannot think clearly and cannot do all the things they really would like to do or need to do.

The second key concept the children learn in C-Session 3 (and C-Session 4) is to manage their anxiety symptoms by using the Stop sign and three cognitive coping strategies, referred to as the Trick Stoppers, which include, Ignore Sneaky Fears, Think Brave Thoughts, and Talk to an Adult.

Prior to the start of C-Session 3, the child group therapists determine their specific roles in the session. At the appropriate start time, at least two child and/or parent group therapists greet parents and children in the waiting area and direct the children to the child group room and the parents to the parent group room. Most children are comfortable about separation by C-Session 3; however, child group therapists are ready to intervene if necessary. As seen in Table 9.2, there are six parts to C-Session 3.

9.3.1 Part One of C-Session 3

Part one of C-Session 3 (Circle Time) begins when all the children are in the child group room and takes five to ten minutes to complete. The first few minutes of part one follow the consistent protocol used to begin each C-Session as outlined in

Sect. 8.5.1, which includes distribution of name tags and spending a minute or two asking the children if they wish to share things about their time since the last session. The child group therapist taking the lead for this portion of the session:

1. Asks if the children remember Leo the Lion and what Leo learned in the story chapters to date (i.e., how to do a Body Scan to be a Feeling Catcher and use Spaghetti Arms and Toes, Balloon Breathing, and Imagery to be the Boss of his Body), and writes these down on the flip chart or white board.
2. Asks if the children have practiced doing Body Scans, Spaghetti Arms and Toes, Balloon Breathing, and Imagery, and provides stickers or other reinforcements, as well as verbal praise, to those who practiced doing Body Scans and relaxation strategies.
3. Practices (briefly) each of the three relaxation strategies with the children, using the scripts for Spaghetti Arms and Toes (Sect. 8.4.4.4), Balloon Breathing (Sect. 8.5.3.2), and Imagery (Sect. 8.5.3.3), dimming the lights if feasible; the child group therapists ensure that the children use the correct techniques, providing support and direction as needed.
4. Expresses the importance of practicing How to Be a Feeling Catcher by doing a Body Scan and practicing each relaxation strategy every single day so that they can be really good at being a Feeling Catcher and being the Boss of their Body, just like Leo the Lion in the story.

The puppets are then distributed and each child chooses a puppet to hold during the Story Time.

9.3.2   Part Two of C-Session 3

As seen in Table 9.2, part two of C-Session 3 (Story Time and discussion of story) takes about ten minutes to complete and consists of reading and discussing Story Chap. 3 of the children's story section of *Taming Sneaky Fears—Leo the Lion's story of bravery & Inside Leo's den: The workbook* (Benoit & Monga, 2018a, b). The child group therapist taking the lead for reading the story reads Story Chap. 3 with a lively and engaging voice and animated facial expressions, while showing the illustrations. The Sneaky Fears puppets are hidden from the children until one of the other child group therapists playing the role of Sneaky Fears makes them suddenly pop out when they make their appearance in the story, and reads Sneaky Fears' words in the story with a snarling (and somewhat scary) voice.

9.3.2.1   Story Discussion

In Story Chap. 3, Leo the Lion attends the Bravery Club where he meets other animals who feel nervous, scared or shy just like he does. Leo meets Ellie the Elephant, another main story character, who is afraid of heights and of making mistakes. Leo identifies and names Sneaky Fears (externalizes his anxiety) and begins to learn a number of strategies to help him tame his Sneaky Fears. After the story is read, the child group therapist leading the story discussion (three to four minutes in duration) asks if the children liked the story, then asks what happened to Leo the Lion in the story (awaits responses such as Leo the Lion went to a Bravery Club, Leo met other animals who felt scared and nervous just like him, Leo used Spaghetti Arms and Toes, Balloon Breathing, and Imagery to be the Boss of his Body and unsqueeze his throat and unstick his voice, Leo the Lion learned that Sneaky Fears were real tricksters who play Tricks on his brain and one of their Tricks is Not Telling the Truth, and Leo the Lion learned the first two Trick Stoppers, Ignore Sneaky Fears and Think Brave Thoughts).

Before moving on to part three, the puppets are returned to the container/cupboard.

9.3.3   Part Three of C-Session 3

Part three of C-Session 3 (How to Be a Trick Catcher and How to Be the Boss of My Brain) takes about 15 minutes to complete and involves discussing with the children aspects of the story to help them understand the concept of Sneaky Fears, the annoying twin jackal puppets that keep bothering Leo (externalization of anxiety) by playing Tricks (cognitive distortions) on Leo's brain.

9.3.3.1   How to Be a Trick Catcher

The lead child group therapist for this portion of the session:

1. Explains that Sneaky Fears are real tricksters and that in order to be the Boss of their Brain, children have to 'catch' the Tricks that Sneaky Fears play and become Trick Catchers.
2. Describes that Sneaky Fears' first Trick is Not Telling the Truth. In the story, Sneaky Fears made Leo the Lion think that his voice would sound funny and that everyone would laugh at him if he used his roar, but that was not true because Leo's mom and dad told him his roar (or voice) sounded great and later, when Leo said, "Got you, Sneaky Fears" at the Bravery Club, no one laughed at him, thus proving to Leo that Sneaky Fears were Not Telling the Truth.
3. Explains that when children feel scared or nervous or some other yucky feeling, it usually means that Sneaky Fears are playing Tricks on their brain, but when children become Trick Catchers and 'catch' (or recognize) the Tricks that Sneaky Fears play, they become the Boss of their Brain.

While describing these concepts, the lead child group therapist writes 'Sneaky Fears' Tricks' in large block letters on the whiteboard (or flip chart) and 'Not Telling the Truth' underneath.

9.3.3.2 How to Use the Stop Sign

The lead child group therapist goes on to describe how to use the Stop sign:

1. Explains that when Sneaky Fears play Tricks on children's brain, one thing children can do is to imagine a big red Stop sign.
2. Asks the children for their suggestions as to what a Stop sign looks like; describes and draws on a white board (or flip chart) the funny (octagonal) shape, the red color of a Stop sign, and the big white letters of the word Stop.
3. Describes that by making their brain imagine and think of a big red Stop sign with its funny (octagonal) shape, its red color, and the big white letters of the word Stop, children keep their brain so busy thinking about the Stop sign that their brain has no time to pay attention to Sneaky Fears; so their brain has no time to think of the scary thoughts that Sneaky Fears are trying to sneak into their brain; that way, children become the Boss of their Brain.
4. Indicates that thinking of the Stop sign also reminds children to Stop and think of using Spaghetti Arms and Toes, Balloon Breathing, or Imagery to calm their body down and Be the Boss of their Body.

9.3.3.3 How to Use the First Two Trick Stoppers

The lead child group therapist goes on to describe how to use the first two Trick Stoppers (Ignore Sneaky Fears and Think Brave Thoughts):

1. Reviews that when children calm their body down by using Spaghetti Arms and Toes, Balloon Breathing, and Imagery, they become the Boss of their Body.
2. Reminds the children that after they calm their body down, it is easier for them to think clearly so that they can Be the Boss of their Brain, use the Stop sign, and 'catch' Sneaky Fears' Tricks.
3. Discusses that children can use the two Trick Stoppers Leo the Lion learned in the story today, Ignore Sneaky Fears or Think Brave Thoughts to tame Sneaky Fears.
4. Explains that when they Ignore or don't listen to Sneaky Fears and instead think Brave Thoughts, they become the Boss of their Brain.
5. Describes that, just like Leo the Lion learned in the story, Ignore Sneaky Fears and Think Brave Thoughts are very powerful Trick Stoppers.
6. Shares that an example of Think Brave Thoughts is thinking, 'I can do it!'

9.3.4 Part Four of C-Session 3

As seen in Table 9.2, part four of C-Session 3 is Craft Time, follows the format outlined in Sect. 8.4.5.1, and takes about ten minutes to complete. One of the child group therapists leads the craft activity by explaining what is required and demonstrating what to draw on the white board (or flip chart) as needed. The other child group therapists distribute the two workbooks, ensure that the children use the correct page of each workbook, and go from child to child to provide support and direction as needed. Craft Time for C-Session 3 has two drawings:

1. The first drawing is found on page 3 of the Supplementary Child Workbook. The lead child group therapist refers back to the Stop sign that was drawn on the white board or flip chart (described in Sect. 9.4.3.2) and then asks the children to draw a Stop sign with the letters Stop in it and color the surrounding area red, leaving the letters white.
2. The second drawing is found on page 68 of the workbook section of *Taming Sneaky Fears—Leo the Lion's story of bravery & Inside Leo's den: The workbook* (Benoit & Monga, 2018a, b). Children draw a picture of themselves using the first two Trick Stoppers, Ignore Sneaky Fears and Think Brave Thoughts. To illustrate 'Ignore Sneaky Fears,' the lead child group therapist could suggest and draw on the white board (or flip chart) a picture of Sneaky Fears (the jackal puppets) with a large X over Sneaky Fears or simply a large X on the page to help children remember to Ignore Sneaky Fears. To illustrate 'Think Brave Thoughts,' the lead child group therapist could suggest or draw a picture of a child with a thought bubble that says, 'I can do it!'[4]

9.3.5 Part Five of C-Session 3

As seen in Table 9.2, part five of C-Session 3 is Snack Time and follows the protocol outlined in Sect. 8.4.6.1.

9.3.6 Part Six of C-Session 3

As seen in Table 9.2, part six of C-Session 3 is wrap up and follows the protocol outlined in Sect. 8.4.7.1.

---

[4]The workbook section of the *Taming Sneaky Fears—Leo the Lion's story of bravery & Inside Leo's den: The workbook* (Benoit & Monga, 2018a, b) contains a number of other drawings that children could do; however, due to time constraints of the group sessions, these drawings are not done in the group (during the parent group sessions and at the final Session 8 (graduation), parents are informed that there are additional drawings that they could encourage their children to do to help the children further integrate what they have learned during the group program).

Table 9.3 Outline of C-Session 4 (excerpt from Table 6.4)

Session[a]	Child group	
	Minutes	
4	5–10	Circle Time—review of events that might have happened to the children since the last session, topics covered during the previous session, and relaxation strategies
	10	Story Time—Chap. 4 of children's story[b] and discussion of story
	15	How to Be a Trick Catcher • Trick #2: Exaggerating • Trick #3: Only Showing the Bad Things How to be the Boss of My Brain • Use the Trick Stopper – Talk to an Adult
	10	Craft Time
	5	Snack Time
	<1	Wrap up
	*Child group therapists meet with each child's parent(s) for five minutes **at the end of Session 4** and (as needed) **immediately prior to the beginning of Session 5** to receive and provide feedback on each child's progress*	

[a]45- to 50-minute session; [b]Children's story section of *Taming Sneaky Fears—Leo the Lion's story of bravery & Inside Leo's den: The workbook* (Benoit & Monga, 2018a, b); <: less than

9.4 Step-by-Step Guidelines to Implement C-Session 4[5]

C-Session 4 continues to teach children how to manage their anxiety by using various cognitive coping strategies. In C-Session 4, the children learn two more of Sneaky Fears' Tricks, Exaggerating and Only Showing the Bad Things. Additionally, the children learn that when they use the Trick Stopper Talk to an Adult, they make Sneaky Fears weaker. By sharing or talking about their fears and worries with trusted adults, such as parents, relatives, teachers, coaches, etc., greater support and problem solving can take place, thereby allowing children to be the Boss of their Brain.

As with other C-Sessions, prior to the start of C-Session 4, the child group therapists decide their respective roles in the session. At the appropriate start time, at least two child and/or parent group therapists go to the waiting room and direct the parents and children to the parent and child group rooms. As seen in Table 9.3, there are six parts to C-Session 4.

---

[5]Session 4 is the mid-point of the Taming Sneaky Fears program and at the end of Session 4, the child group therapists start to meet with each child's parent(s) to provide and receive feedback on the child's progress. Section 11.2 provides details about the parent feedback component to the program, which the child group therapists read prior to C-Session 4.

9.4.1   Part One of C-Session 4

Part one of C-Session 4 (Circle Time—review of events that might have occurred to the children since the last session, review and practice of relaxation strategies) follows the protocol outline in Sect. 9.3.1. The child group therapist leading Circle Time reviews the concepts children learned at C-Session 3 by:

1. Asking the children if they remember Sneaky Fears and how sneaky Sneaky Fears can be (most children are quite enamored by Sneaky Fears and can get quite excited talking about the character).
2. Reminding the children that learning How to Be the Boss of their Brain will help them tame Sneaky Fears.
3. Reviewing How to Be a Trick Catcher in order to catch the Tricks that Sneaky Fears play.
4. Reiterating that when children feel scared or nervous or some other yucky feeling it usually means that Sneaky Fears are playing Tricks on their brain, but when children become Trick Catchers and 'catch' (or recognize) the Tricks that Sneaky Fears play, children (and not Sneaky Fears) become the Boss of their Brain.
4. Explaining that Sneaky Fears' first Trick is Not Telling the Truth.
5. Reviewing how and why to use the Stop sign.
6. Reminding the children that Ignore Sneaky Fears and Think Brave Thoughts are the first two Trick Stoppers.

The lead child group therapist writes these key concepts down on the white board (or flip chart) as the review takes place.

The puppets are then distributed and each child selects a puppet to hold on to for Story Time (and discussion of the story).

9.4.2   Part Two of C-Session 4

Part two of C-Session 4 (Story Time and discussion of story) takes about ten minutes to complete. The child group therapist leading this part begins with a brief discussion and explanation of what Exaggerating means by describing exaggerating as making something bigger than it really is. The lead child group therapist could use the example of saying 'I'm so hungry that I could eat a hundred hotdogs,' and then asking the children if it is possible to eat a hundred hotdogs. Children quickly recognize that eating a hundred hotdogs is not possible as it is too many hotdogs to eat and thereby understand that the therapist is Exaggerating. Other examples that explain the concept of exaggeration could be 'I'm so thirsty I could drink a hundred cans of pop' or 'I think I might have a million cavities.'

Once the children understand the concept of Exaggerating, the lead child group therapist reads Story Chap. 4 of *Taming Sneaky Fears—Leo the Lion's story of bravery & Inside Leo's den: The workbook* (Benoit & Monga, 2018a, b) with a lively and engaging voice and animated facial expressions, while showing the illustrations. Again, one of the child group therapists plays the role of Sneaky Fears, reading Sneaky Fears' words in the story with a snarling (and somewhat scary) voice.

9.4.2.1 Story Discussion

After the story is read, the child group therapist leading the story discussion (three to four minutes in duration) asks if the children liked the story and what happened to Leo the Lion in the story. The lead child group therapist awaits responses such as Leo the Lion learned two more of Sneaky Fears' Tricks (Exaggerating and Only Showing the Bad Things) and another powerful Trick Stopper (Talk to an Adult).

Before moving on to part three, the puppets are returned to the container.

9.4.3 Part Three of C-Session 4

Part three of C-Session 4 (How to Be a Trick Catcher and How to Be the Boss of My Brain) takes about 15 minutes to complete and involves discussing with the children aspects of the story to help them understand Sneaky Fears' two other Tricks: Exaggerating and Only Showing the Bad Things, and the third Trick Stopper, Talk to an Adult. The lead child group therapist for this portion of Session 4:

1. Explains that although Sneaky Fears can be tricksters, Sneaky Fears only know three Tricks.
2. Reviews and highlights how Leo the Lion was a Trick Catcher and caught (or recognized) two more of Sneaky Fears' Tricks; Leo the Lion realized that his voice could not be stuck in his throat forever and figured out that Sneaky Fears were Exaggerating; Leo the Lion also figured out that Sneaky Fears were Only Showing the Bad Things as Sneaky Fears did not want Leo to see any of the good things about being friends with Ellie the Elephant (e.g., how much fun Leo would have with Ellie).
3. Describes the third Trick Stopper, Talk to an Adult, and explains how Sneaky Fears got weaker when Leo the Lion used this Trick Stopper, Talk to an Adult.
4. Encourages children to think of various adults at home (e.g., parents, grandparents, other important caregivers) and at school (e.g., teachers, principal, coaches) that children could talk to when their own Sneaky Fears are bothering them and making them feel nervous or scared) and writes these down on the whiteboard (or flip chart).

9.4.4   Part Four of C-Session 4

As seen in Table 9.3, part four of C-Session 4 is Craft Time, follows the format outlined in Sect. 8.4.5.1, and takes about ten minutes to complete.

One of the child group therapists leads the craft activity by explaining what is required and demonstrating what to draw on the white board (or flip chart) as needed. The other child group therapists distribute *Taming Sneaky Fears—Leo the Lion's story of bravery & Inside Leo's den: The workbook* (Benoit & Monga, 2018a, b), which contains the drawings the children do for C-Session 4. The other child group therapists ensure that the children are on the correct page for each craft and go from child to child to provide support and direction as needed. Craft Time for C-Session 4 has three drawings for the children to make in the workbook section of *Taming Sneaky Fears—Leo the Lion's story of bravery & Inside Leo's den: The workbook* (Benoit & Monga, 2018a, b):

1. The first drawing is on page 71. The children draw a picture of the Trick Exaggerating. For this, the lead child group therapist could draw a number of ice cream cones, or a number of cookies (or an excessive number of some other easy-to-draw item) on the white board (or flip chart) to demonstrate that the idea that Exaggerating is to make something bigger or worse than it is—as in, 'I'm so hungry I could eat 100 cookies'.
2. The second drawing is at the top of page 73. The children draw a picture of themselves using the third Trick Stopper, Talk to an Adult. The lead child group therapist could draw on the white board (or flip chart) a child (or stick figure) talking to an adult (a larger stick figure that could be labeled mom, dad, teacher, etc.)
3. The third drawing is found on page 74. The children list (or draw pictures of) other trusted adults to whom they can talk when they use their Trick Stopper Talk to an Adult. The lead child group therapist could list or draw trusted adults such as grandparents, teachers, principal, coaches, or other adults the children trust while the other child group therapists assist the children as needed.[6]

---

[6]The workbook section of *Taming Sneaky Fears—Leo the Lion's story of bravery & Inside Leo's den: The workbook* (Benoit & Monga, 2018a, b) contains a number of other drawings that children could do; however, due to time constraints of the group sessions, these drawings are not done in the group (during the parent group sessions and at the final Session 8 (graduation), parents are informed that there are additional drawings that they could encourage their children to do to help the children further integrate what they have learned during the group program).

9.4.5 Part Five of C-Session 4

As seen in Table 9.3, part five of C-Session 4 is Snack Time and follows the protocol outlined in Sect. 8.4.6.1.

9.4.6 Part Six of C-Session 4

As seen in Table 9.3, part six of C-Session 4 is wrap up and follows the protocol outlined in Sect. 8.4.7.1.

References

Benoit, D., & Monga, S. (2018a). *Apprivoiser les Peurs-pas-fines—L'histoire de bravoure de Léo le lionceau & Dans la tanière de Léo: Le cahier de travail*. Victoria, British Columbia: FriesenPress.
Benoit, D., & Monga, S. (2018b). *Taming Sneaky Fears—Leo the Lion's story of bravery & Inside Leo's den: The workbook*. Victoria, British Columbia: FriesenPress.

Chapter 10
The Taming Sneaky Fears Program: How to Climb Bravery Ladders and How to Manage Excessive Worries

10.1 Overview and Rationale

In the Taming Sneaky Fears program, the abstract concept of progressive desensitization or gradual exposure is made concrete by referring to it as How to Climb Bravery Ladders. Children learn that by climbing one small step of a Bravery Ladder at a time, they go from behaving in ways that show they are feeling and looking nervous or scared of a situation (at the bottom of the Bravery Ladder) to behaving in ways that show they are feeling and looking brave in that same situation (at the top of the Bravery Ladder). The concept of How to Climb Bravery Ladders to overcome fears is introduced to the parents in one session (P-Session 3) and to the children in two sessions (C-Sessions 6 and 7). In P-Session 3 and subsequent sessions, parents learn that progressive desensitization or gradual exposure (How to Climb Bravery Ladders) is an appropriate strategy for overcoming specific phobias and many other fears such as being away from caregivers (separation anxiety), making mistakes (perfectionism), being seen and heard speaking (selective mutism), and being in the spotlight, judged, or doing something embarrassing (social anxiety). In P-Session 3, parents learn additional strategies for managing their young children's excessive worries (as seen in generalized anxiety disorder).

10.2 Step-by-Step Guidelines to Implement P-Session 3

Prior to the start of P-Session 3, the parent group therapists obtain from the child group therapists a list of available five-minute appointment times for parents to meet with the child group therapists immediately after P-Session 4 is over or immediately prior to the start of P-Session 5 (the number of appointment times depends on the number of child group therapists available to provide and receive the feedback and the number of children participating in the group). Also prior to the start of

© Springer Nature Switzerland AG 2018
S. Monga and D. Benoit, *Assessing and Treating Anxiety Disorders in Young Children*, https://doi.org/10.1007/978-3-030-04939-3_10

Table 10.1 Outline of P-Session 3 (excerpt from Table 6.4)

Session[a]	Parent group	
	Minutes	
3	5–10	Scheduling of parent feedback meetings with the child group therapists Brave moments and effective praise
	5–10	Review of other tasks
	30–40	How to Climb Bravery Ladders (to overcome fears) How to manage excessive worries
	<1	Wrap up

[a]45- to 50-minute session; <: less than

P-Session 3, the parent group therapists determine which parent group therapists are in charge of each specific part of P-Session 3 and ensure that all the materials needed (Table 6.3) are available in the parent group room.

As P-Session 3 is about to start, at least two child and/or parent group therapists go to the waiting area to greet all parents and children and bring them to their respective room.[1]

As seen in Table 10.1, P-Session 3 is divided into four parts.

10.2.1 Part One of P-Session 3

As the parents enter the parent group room, one of the parent group therapists welcomes them and invites them to take their name tag from the table and put it on as they make themselves comfortable. If parents are in charge of bringing the snack for the child group session, the lead parent group therapist thanks the parent who brought the snack and reminds the parents of which parent is in charge of bringing the children's snack for the next session. The parent group therapists then proceed with part one of P-Session 3 (scheduling of feedback meetings with the child group therapists and brave moments and effective praise), which, as seen in Table 10.1, takes 5–10 minutes to complete.

The lead parent group therapist circulates the list of appointment times the child group therapists provided prior to the start of P-Session 3 and explains to the parents that the next session (Session 4) is the mid-point in the Taming Sneaky Fears program and a child group therapist will meet with each of the children's parents for about five minutes immediately after Session 4 or immediately before Session 5 begins. The lead parent group therapist asks the parents to write their name down next to the appointment date and time they wish to attend and provides a copy of the list to the child group therapists at the end of P-Session 3 (Note: It is useful for the parent group

---

[1]If parents are in charge of bringing the snacks for the child group sessions, it is typically at that moment that the parent who brings the snack gives it to one of the child group therapists.

therapists to keep the list as they will need to remind the parents of their appointment dates and times during Session 4).

The parent group therapist leading this part of P-Session 3 asks two or three parents to volunteer examples of brave moments they noticed in their children since the previous session and how they provided effective praise. As done in previous P-Sessions (Sect. 8.3.2), the lead parent group therapist encourages parent engagement by:

1. Inviting supportive comments from other parents on what the parents volunteering examples did well when providing effective praise and what they could have done differently to provide even more effective praise.
2. Asking parents to review the three main characteristics of effective praise (i.e., start praise with a '*You*' statement, focus on the *specific behavior* displayed by the child, provide praise *as soon as possible* after the display of the brave behavior).
3. Asking parents to explain the rationale for identifying brave moments and providing effective praise (i.e., the more one pays attention to a behavior, the more likely the behavior is to be repeated).

As done in previous P-Sessions, throughout this part, the parent group therapists actively provide constructive feedback to the parents who volunteer examples and comments. The parent group therapists remind the parents that focusing on brave moments and providing effective praise are tasks throughout the program (and ideally, would continue even after the Taming Sneaky Fears program is completed).

10.2.2 Part Two of P-Session 3

As seen in Table 10.1, part two of P-Session 3 (review of other tasks) takes five to ten minutes to complete. One parent group therapist takes the lead for this part and completes the following tasks:

1. Asks the parents to volunteer how they encouraged their children to practice doing Body Scans and the relaxation strategies.
2. Promotes parent engagement by inviting comments on what the parents volunteering examples did well when they encouraged their children to practice doing Body Scans (and/or charades) and the relaxation strategies, and what they could do if their children show resistance to doing Body Scans (and/or charades) and practicing the relaxation strategies.
3. Reiterates the importance for children to practice the various relaxation strategies at least twice a day, for at least five minutes each time, when they are calm and relaxed, in order to master the strategies so they will work better when the children need them (as mentioned in the list from the Parent Session 3 Tasks section of the Parent Manual[2]); parents can use the practice charts provided in the Parent Manual (Fig. 14 for Spaghetti Arms and Toes, Fig. 15 for Balloon Breathing,

---

[2]The Parent Manual is provided as one of the Supplementary Materials in Chap. 6.

and Fig. 16 for Balloon Breathing and Imagery together) or make their own if they wish.

4. Reminds the parents that the children receive stickers as rewards during the child group sessions if they report having practiced the relaxation strategies between sessions.

5. Mentions to the parents that the children practice each relaxation strategy at the beginning of each child session, under the child group therapists' supervision.

10.2.3   Part Three of P-Session 3

Part three of P-Session 3 (How to Climb Bravery Ladders and how to manage excessive worries) takes 30 to 40 minutes to complete. It is content heavy and the parent group therapists mention this to the parents and ensure to pace themselves so they can cover all the materials during the allotted time.

10.2.3.1   How to Climb Bravery Ladders

To begin part three of P-Session 3, the parent group therapist leading this portion:

1. Mentions to the parents that today in the children's group, the children:

   a. Meet Sneaky Fears.
   b. Learn about Sneaky Fears' first Trick, Not Telling the Truth.
   c. Learn How to Be the Boss of My Brain by using the Stop sign and the first two Trick Stoppers, Ignore Sneaky Fears and Think Brave Thoughts.

2. Shows the children's workbooks, including the workbook section of *Taming Sneaky Fears—Leo the Lion's story of bravery & Inside Leo's den: The workbook* (Benoit & Monga, 2018a, b) and the Supplementary Child Workbook[3] to the parents and points out the drawings the children are doing during today's Session 3: the Stop sign and the first two Trick Stoppers, Ignore Sneaky Fears and Think Brave Thoughts.

3. Reminds the parents that, as mentioned in previous sessions, they do not have the children's workbooks in their possession, as these are kept with the child group therapists until 'graduation' (Session 8) when the children's workbooks are given to the children to take home; mentions to the parent that the workbook section of *Taming Sneaky Fears—Leo the Lion's story of bravery & Inside Leo's den: The workbook* (Benoit & Monga, 2018a, b) contains more activities the children could do than time allows in the group sessions, so at the end of the group program, parents could complete these additional activities with the children to help them further integrate the concepts they have learned during the group sessions.

---

[3]The Supplementary Child Workbook is provided as one of the Supplementary Materials in Chap. 6.

4. Reiterates the importance for parents to ensure that their children master the concepts of being Feeling Catchers and doing Body Scans, and use the correct techniques when doing Spaghetti Arms and Toes, Balloon Breathing, and Imagery (and reiterates the need for children to practice each relaxation strategy for at least five minutes, every day, when they are relaxed and do not need the relaxation strategy), as mentioned in the tasks for P-Session 3.
5. Directs the parents to Fig. 21 of the Parent Manual (and points out where Fig. 21 is located), while using the laminated copy of Fig. 3 from the Parent Manual that illustrates the overlap between traditional CBT and the Taming Sneaky Fears program to remind parents that during Session 1, the focus was on the 'Feeling' component of the cognitive triangle, during the last session the focus was on the 'Thought' component of the cognitive triangle, and today the focus of our session is on the 'Behavior' component of the cognitive triangle.
6. Explains the rationale for using progressive desensitization or gradual exposure (or climbing Bravery Ladders) to overcome specific fears:

    a. Two techniques can be used to help children, adolescents, and adults overcome their fears:
        i.   Flooding, which could look something like placing someone who has a strong fear of dogs in the close proximity of a dog, for two or three hours, until the person's anxiety decreases; understandably, flooding can create much distress and is not a technique that is typically used with young children.
        ii. Progressive desensitization or gradual exposure, which could look something like having someone who has a strong fear of dogs *gradually, over time,* approach a dog (e.g., by a couple of feet each day, so that over a period of days or weeks the person is close enough to pet the dog); this technique is usually preferred with young children as it typically creates less distress in the child than flooding; it is a technique that consists of taking small, manageable steps to reach a goal that would usually be unreachable without steps (much like ladders have steps to help someone climb, one step at a time, to reach something that would otherwise be out of reach); in the Taming Sneaky Fears program, the expression *Climbing My Bravery Ladders* refers to this technique.
    b. Points out that the concept of a Bravery Ladder helps young children picture themselves slowly climbing up the steps of their Bravery Ladder, i.e., becoming brave and overcoming their fears, one small step at a time, much like one of the main story characters, Ellie the Elephant, does in the story that is read in the child group; young children can picture starting at the bottom of the ladder (or where they are now, i.e., behaving in a way that shows they are shy, nervous, or scared of a specific object or situation), climbing one step at a time (like Ellie the Elephant does in the story) all the way up the top step of

the ladder (or where they want to be, i.e., behaving in a way that shows they are brave or not shy, nervous, or scared of that object or situation anymore).

7. Explains that examples of specific fears that can be tackled with Bravery Ladders include fear of making mistakes (perfectionism), fear of being away from a parent (separation anxiety), fear of being seen and heard speaking (selective mutism), fear of being in the spotlight, judged, or doing something embarrassing (social anxiety), fear of dogs (or other animals or insects), fear of the dark, fear of heights, etc.

8. Directs the parents' attention to the section of the Parent Manual that describes the Essential Ingredients for Success with Bravery Ladders (and points out where the parents can find this information in their Parent Manual); the parent group therapist goes over this information in detail, point by point, asking the parents to follow along.

9. Asks the parents to look at the titles of the next subsections in the Parent Manual, while indicating the page numbers where this information is located (i.e., General Principles and Example of Selective Mutism, Example of Excessive Shyness, Examples of Specific Phobia/Separation Anxiety, Example of Perfectionism) and mentions to the parents that depending on what their child's fears are, they could choose to focus on a specific subsection.[4]

10. Directs the parents' attention to the section that pertains to How to Implement Bravery Ladders (including at school); the parent group therapist does not read this section in detail, and only emphasizes that this section provides parents and teachers (or other adults implementing Bravely Ladders) with specific ideas about how to implement Bravery Ladders.

11. Reminds the parents that as seen in item 8 of the What to Do to Help list (Fig. 4 of the Parent Manual), the Taming Sneaky Fears program encourages parents to remind their children How to Climb Bravery Ladders to show that they are becoming brave.

12. Mentions that as a task after today's session, parents are asked to start developing a Bravery Ladder for their children to climb, using Fig. 28 of the Parent Manual (and the Bravery Ladder they work on will be discussed during an upcoming session if they wish).

13. Directs the parents' attention to the section of the Parent Manual that focuses on 'Supportively Push Young Anxious Children Past Their Fears,' as well as the corresponding item 9 of the What to Do to Help list (Fig. 4 of the Parent Manual), and reviews the information.

---

[4]The parent group therapist leading this part of P-Session 3 is aware of the children's anxiety diagnoses and tailors the information provided to the parents in the group to address the specific fears or phobias that the children exhibit. For example, if at least one child in the group has selective mutism, the parent group therapist carefully reviews the subsection on General Principles and Example of Selective Mutism.

10.2.3.2   How to Manage Excessive Worries

The parent group therapist leading this part:

1. Directs the parents' attention to the section of the Parent Manual that focuses on How to Manage Excessive Worries and highlights that this represents item 10 of the What to Do to Help list (Fig. 4 of the Parent Manual).
2. Describes Dr. Huebner's recommended strategies:

   a. Containment of worries.
   b. Externalization.
   c. Competing demands.

   The description is detailed if there is at least one child in the group who worries excessively, but the description can be more cursory if no child in the group worries excessively.
3. If possible, uses a copy of Dr. Huebner's workbook, *What to do when you worry too much* during the discussion of Dr. Huebner's recommended strategies (e.g., shows the illustration of the Worry Box and the page in Dr. Huebner's workbook where the children draw a picture of the worry bullies to *externalize* anxiety).
4. Reminds parents that in the Taming Sneaky Fears program, anxiety is *externalized* by referring to it as Sneaky Fears.

10.2.3.3   Parent Session 3 Tasks

The parent group therapist leading this part:

1. Briefly reviews the tasks until the next session.
2. Reminds the parents that some of them will meet with a child group therapist at the end of the next session (Session 4, or just before the beginning of Session 5) to receive feedback on how their children are doing in the group; this will also be the opportunity for parents to provide an update on how they think their children are doing outside of the group.

10.2.4   Part Four of P-Session 3

Part four of P-Session 3 (wrap up) takes 30–60 seconds to complete and as mentioned in the protocols of previous P-Sessions (e.g., Sect. 8.3.4), it starts when one of the child group therapists knocks at the door and enters the parent group room to provide a ten-second summary of the topic(s) covered during the child session that day. As soon as the child group therapist departs, the lead parent therapist thanks the parents for their attention and cooperation during today's session, and reminds parents:

1. That the child group therapist coming in is the signal for the parent group session to end promptly as the children are ready to be picked up.

2. To remove their name tags and place them on the table as these are re-used at each session.
3. To go to the children's group room to pick up their children.

10.3   Step-by-Step Guidelines to Implement C-Session 6

In C-Session 6, the concept of How to Climb a Bravery Ladder is introduced to the children. The key concept the children learn in C-Sessions 6 and 7 is that when they take small baby steps, they can go from where they are now, feeling scared and nervous or shy, to where they would like to be, feeling brave. Given the young age of the children, the children's parents (and not the children) actually build the Bravery Ladders, with the support and guidance of the parent group therapists. Therefore, the main goals of C-Sessions 6 and 7 are to help children understand the purpose of a Bravery Ladder and to get motivated to work with their parent(s) to Climb a Bravery Ladder to become brave (and become gradually less scared and nervous), just like Leo the Lion and Ellie the Elephant did in the story. Children learn that when they are at the bottom of their Bravery Ladder (all nervous and scared), their Sneaky Fears are wild and scary, but when they have climbed to the top of their Bravery Ladder, they have become brave and have tamed their Sneaky Fears, just like Leo the Lion and Ellie the Elephant did in the story.

As usual, before C-Session 6 begins, the child group therapists decide amongst themselves what parts of C-Session 6 they each are responsible for covering. At the appropriate start time, at least two child and/or parent group therapists greet parents and children in the waiting area and direct the children to the child group room and the parents to the parent group room. As seen in Table 10.2, there are six parts to C-Session 6.

Table 10.2   Outline of C-Session 6 (excerpt from Table 6.4)

Session[a]	Child group	
	Minutes	
6	5–10	Circle time—review of events that might have happened to the children since the last session, topics covered in the previous session, and relaxation strategies
	10	Story time—Chap. 6 of the children's story[b] and discussion of story
	15	How to Climb Bravery Ladders
	10	Craft Time
	5	Snack Time
	<1	Wrap up

[a]45- to 50-minute session; [b]Children's story section of *Taming Sneaky Fears—Leo the Lion's story of bravery & Inside Leo's den: The workbook* (Benoit & Monga, 2018a, b); <: less than

10.3.1 Part One of C-Session 6

Part one of C-Session 6 (Circle Time) takes 5–10 minutes to complete and begins with the usual protocol of welcoming the children, distributing name tags, discussing events or activities children wish to share with others, asking children if they practiced Spaghetti Arms and Toes and Balloon Breathing (and providing stickers or other reinforcements for practicing), and practicing Spaghetti Arms and Toes, Balloon Breathing, and Imagery for a few minutes (while dimming the lights, if feasible; the child group therapists ensure that the children use the correct techniques and provide support and direction as needed).

The child group therapist taking the lead for this part of the session:

1. Reviews the concept of a Feeling Thermometer and how it measures whether one is feeling just a little nervous (like a 1 or 2 on the Feeling Thermometer), or feeling more nervous and scared (like at a 5 or 6), or the most scared or nervous they have ever felt (like at a 9 or 10).
2. Reminds the children that when they are feeling at a 5 or higher on their Feeling Thermometer, that means Sneaky Fears are playing Tricks on their brain and if they use Spaghetti Arms and Toes, Balloon Breathing, or Imagery when their Feeling Thermometer is at a 5 or higher, they can calm their body down and become the Boss of their Body.
3. Reviews how to use the Stop sign.
4. Asks the children to name the three Tricks that Sneaky Fears play (Not Telling the Truth, Exaggerating, and Only Showing the Bad Things) and the three Trick Stoppers (Ignore Sneaky Fears, Think Brave Thoughts, and Talk to an Adult), while encouraging the children to call out the various Tricks and Trick Stoppers and making sure to write these down on the white board (or flip chart).
5. Encourages the children to share examples of what Tricks their own Sneaky Fears have played on their brain since the last session and what Trick Stoppers they used to start taming their Sneaky Fears.

The puppets are then distributed and each child chooses a puppet to hold during part two of the session.

10.3.2 Part Two of C-Session 6

As seen in Table 10.2, part two of C-Session 6 (Story Time and discussion of story) takes about 10 minutes to complete. The child group therapist leading this portion of the session reads Story Chap. 6 of *Taming Sneaky Fears—Leo the Lion's story of bravery & Inside Leo's den: The workbook* (Benoit & Monga, 2018a, b) with a lively and engaging voice and animated facial expressions while showing the illustrations. One of the child group therapists plays the role of Ellie the Elephant's own Sneaky Fears, Missy Mistake, reading Missy Mistake's words in the story with a screeching (and somewhat scary) voice.

10.3.2.1   Story Discussion

After Story Chap. 6 is read, the child group therapist leading the story discussion (three to four minutes in duration) asks:

1. If the children liked the story.
2. Who is Missy Mistake? (Ellie has a Sneaky Fears that she calls Missy Mistake).
3. What happened to Leo and Ellie in the story? (Leo sees a present on the top of Ellie's bunk bed; Leo learns that Ellie is too afraid to climb the ladder to get the present; Leo helps Ellie to be the Boss of her Body and Brain and climb the first two steps of the ladder of her bunk bed).

   Before moving on to part three, the puppets are returned to the puppet container.

10.3.3   Part Three of C-Session 6

As seen in Table 10.2, part three of C-Session 6 (How to Climb Bravery Ladders) takes about 15 minutes to complete and involves discussing aspects of the story to help the children understand the concept of How to Climb a Bravery Ladder. The child group therapist leading this portion of the session:

1. Explains that a Bravery Ladder helps children take little baby steps, one at a time, to go from where they are now at the bottom of the ladder, feeling scared or nervous or shy, to the top of the ladder where they will be brave (and not so scared or nervous or shy anymore).
2. Ensures that the children understand that when they are at the bottom of their Bravery Ladder, they do not feel brave, but when they have climbed all the steps of their Bravery Ladder, they show that they have become really brave and have become the Boss of their Body and the Boss of their Brain.
3. Emphasizes that at the bottom of the Bravery Ladder, Sneaky Fears are wild and the boss, but when children get to the top of their Bravery Ladder, the children are the Boss of their Body and Brain and have tamed Sneaky Fears!
4. Describes that just like Ellie the Elephant in the story, children can choose to climb only one step or climb more than one step of their Bravery Ladder at a time. And just like Ellie the Elephant, children will probably feel really nervous about going up the first step. But just like Ellie the Elephant did in the story, they can use the Feeling Thermometer to measure how scared or nervous they feel and if they feel at a 5 or higher, they can use Spaghetti Arms and Toes, Balloon Breathing, and Imagery to calm their body down so they can keep climbing their Bravery Ladder. Just like Ellie, if they push themselves and climb that first step of their first Bravery Ladder, they are becoming brave.

   When conducting groups with young children who have a diversity of fears, it is neither realistic nor feasible to build, in session, as many specific Bravery Ladders as would be needed to address each and every specific fear that each child has.

Furthermore, the goal of the child group sessions that pertain to Bravery Ladders is not to have the children learn how to *build* a Bravery Ladder, but instead, as mentioned above, the goal is to help the children understand the concept that Climbing a Bravery Ladder, one small step at a time, makes them become increasingly braver and makes their Sneaky Fears increasingly tamer. In the C-sessions devoted to Bravery Ladders, young children learn that a Bravery Ladder (1) has a name that indicates what they are going to do to show that they have become brave when they have climbed to the top of the Bravery Ladder and (2) is made up of four to six different baby steps that they will climb, one at a time, just like Leo the Lion and Ellie the Elephant do in the story.

10.3.3.1 How to Climb a Bravery Ladder for Being Friendly

The child group therapists tailor the contents of part three of C-Session 6 (and C-Session 7) to meet the specific needs of the children in the group. For example, in groups where most children have a number of different fears, the child group therapists use a Bravery Ladder for Being Friendly that is adapted from Fig. 25 of the Parent Manual to include four steps (Section "Groups of Children Who Have Various Fears") to illustrate the key concepts of a Bravery Ladder (as described above). In groups where a large proportion of children have selective mutism and/or social anxiety disorder, the child group therapists use a Bravery Ladder for Being Friendly that is also adapted from Fig. 25 of the Parent Manual and includes six steps (Section "Groups of Children with Selective Mutism and/or Social Anxiety Disorder"). With both groups of children, the child group therapists use a large laminated Bravery Ladder (Fig. 28 of the Parent Manual) with Velcro pieces on each step of the Bravery Ladder and small laminated illustrations (with Velcro at the back of the illustrations) that depict each of the four or six steps of the Bravery Ladder for Being Friendly (as described in Sections "Groups of Children Who Have Various Fears" and "Groups of Children with Selective Mutism and/or Social Anxiety Disorder"). The Velcro pieces on the Bravery Ladder steps and on each illustration allow the therapists and/or children to attach the small laminated illustrations to the large laminated Bravery Ladder.[5]

Groups of Children Who Have Various Fears

The child group therapist leading part three of C-Session 6 with groups of children who have various fears:

---

[5]The large laminated Bravery Ladder used in Sections "Groups of Children Who Have Various Fears" and "Groups of Children with Selective Mutism and/or Social Anxiety Disorder" is a version of Fig. 25 of the Parent Manual with Velcro glued on to each rung and will need to be created prior to the session; while each laminated step is a picture corresponding to the description of the step with Velcro glued on to the back and it too will need to be created prior to the session.

1. Explains and shows, using the large laminated Bravery Ladder with Velcro pieces, that a Bravery Ladder for Being Friendly has four steps (shows the four laminated illustrations that each have a piece of Velcro at the back).
2. Explains that the first step (Step 1) to be friendly is to stay in the room (away from mom or dad) with the person with whom they want to be friendly, and attaches a laminated illustration (with Velcro on the back) of two children standing side by side to the piece of Velcro that is on Step 1 of the Bravery Ladder.
3. Describes that the second step (Step 2) is to face and look at the person with whom they want to be friendly, and attaches a laminated illustration (with Velcro on the back) of a pair of eyes (or of two children facing each other and looking at each other) to the piece of Velcro that is on Step 2 of the Bravery Ladder.
4. Explains that the third step (Step 3) is to smile to the person with whom they want to be friendly, and attaches a laminated illustration (with Velcro on the back) of a face with a big smile (or of two children facing each other and smiling to each other) to the piece of Velcro that is on Step 3 of the Bravery Ladder.
5. Indicates that the fourth and final step (Step 4) of a Bravery Ladder for Being Friendly is to say "Hi" and share their name with the person with whom they want be friendly, and attaches a laminated illustration of two children facing each other with smiles and saying "Hi, my name is____" (a thought bubble could have this phrase). The illustration (with Velcro on the back) is attached to the piece of Velcro on Step 4 of the Bravery Ladder.
6. Removes the four laminated illustrations from the four steps of the Bravery Ladder for Being Friendly and asks the children for help in rebuilding the Bravery Ladder:

    a. Asks the children to call out what each step of the Bravery Ladder is.
    b. Re-attaches the appropriate illustrations on to each of the four steps or asks for volunteers to come up and place each illustration on the appropriate step on the Bravery Ladder, until the Bravery Ladder is complete again.

Groups of Children with Selective Mutism and/or Social Anxiety Disorder

For groups that have a significant number of children with selective mutism and/or social anxiety disorder, Step 4 of the Bravery Ladder for Being Friendly (Section "Groups of Children Who Have Various Fears") above (say "Hi" and share their name with the person with whom they want to be friendly) is broken down into additional steps. The reason for this is that climbing from Step 3 (smile to the person with whom they want to be friendly) to Step 4 (say "Hi" and share their name in a normal volume voice) is too big a step for children with selective mutism and/or social anxiety and therefore requires to be broken into additional steps: say "Hi" and share their name in a whisper voice (Step 4) and say "Hi" and share their name in a quiet or soft voice (Step 5), and say "Hi" and share their name in a normal volume voice (Step 6).

The child group therapist leading this part of the session with groups of children with selective mutism and/or social anxiety disorder:

1. Completes the Steps 1 to 3 of the Bravery Ladder for Being Friendly as described in Section "Groups of Children Who Have Various Fears".
2. Divides Step 4 (from Section "Groups of Children Who Have Various Fears") into additional steps and explains that:

   a. Step 4 is to say "Hi" and share their name with the person with whom they are trying to be friendly, using a *whisper* voice; the lead child group therapist attaches to the piece of Velcro on the fourth step of the Bravery Ladder a laminated illustration (with Velcro on the back) of two children facing each other with smiles and saying "Hi, my name is____" (a thought bubble could have this phrase in small letters depicting a whisper voice).

   b. Step 5 is to increase the voice volume and to say "Hi" and share their name with the person with whom they are trying to be friendly in a *quiet or soft* voice; the lead child group therapist attaches to the piece of Velcro on the fifth step of the Bravery Ladder a laminated illustration (with Velcro on the back) of two children facing each other with smiles and saying "Hi, my name is____" (a thought bubble could have this phrase in slightly bigger letters depicting a quiet or soft voice).

   c. Step 6 is to increase the voice volume to a *normal* volume voice and to say "Hi" and share their name with the person with whom they are trying to be friendly in a *normal volume* voice; the lead child group therapist attaches to the piece of Velcro on the sixth step of the Bravery Ladder a laminated illustration (with Velcro on the back) of two children facing each other with smiles and saying "Hi, my name is____" (a thought bubble could have this phrase in slightly bigger letters depicting a normal volume voice).

3. Removes the six laminated illustrations from the six steps of the Bravery Ladder for Being Friendly and asks the children for help in rebuilding the Bravery Ladder:

   a. Asks the children to call out what each step of the Bravery Ladder is.
   b. Re-attaches the appropriate illustrations on to each of the six steps or asks for volunteers to come up and place each illustration on the appropriate step on the Bravery Ladder, until the Bravery Ladder is complete again.

10.3.4 Part Four of C-Session 6

As seen in Table 10.2, part four of C-Session 6 is Craft Time, follows the format outlined in Sect. 8.4.5.1, and takes about ten minutes to complete. One of the child group therapists leads the craft activity by explaining what is required and demonstrating what to draw on the white board (or flip chart) as needed. The other child group therapists distribute *Taming Sneaky Fears—Leo the Lion's story of bravery & Inside Leo's den: The workbook* (Benoit & Monga, 2018a, b) and ensure that the children are on the correct page (page 80). Craft Time for C-Session 6 has only one component but requires that the child group therapists go from child to child to provide individual attention and assistance to each child.

The lead child group therapist draws a Bravery Ladder on the white board (or flip chart) with two boxes (similar to the illustration on page 80) and asks the children for suggestions of what they are doing currently that demonstrates that they are scared or nervous and draws in the bottom box on the white board (or flip chart) some examples (e.g., not speaking to friends or teachers, sleeping with mom or dad, being afraid of dogs). The lead child group therapist asks the children to draw in the bottom box of the Bravery Ladder a picture of what they do now that shows they are feeling scared and nervous. The other child group therapists provide the necessary individual attention and assistance each child requires to determine what they are doing now that shows that they are scared, nervous, or shy.

The lead child group therapist then asks the children for suggestions of what they will be doing when they are no longer scared or nervous and have become brave, and draws in the top box on the white board (or flip chart) some examples (e.g., saying hi or speaking to friends or teachers, sleeping in their own bed, petting a dog). The lead child group then asks the children to draw in the top box of the Bravery Ladder a picture of what they will do when they have reached the top of their Bravery Ladder and are brave.

The other child group therapists go from child to child to help each child decide what to draw in the two boxes and identify the main theme of his or her Bravery Ladder (e.g., My Bravery Ladder for Using My Normal Voice for Speaking to My Teacher, My Bravery Ladder for Sleeping By Myself in My Bedroom, My Bravery Ladder for Petting My Auntie's Dog). The child group therapist can assist the children in writing the name of each child's Bravery Ladder in the space provided in the banner area of the drawing.

10.3.5 Part Five of C-Session 6

As seen in Table 10.2, part five of C-Session 6 is Snack Time and follows the protocol outlined in Sect. 8.4.6.1. Beginning in C-Session 6, the child group therapists gather information from each child during Snack Time about what they like to do so that some personalized details can be added to each Graduation Certificate as further discussed in Chap. 11.

10.3.6 Part Six of C-Session 6

As seen in Table 10.2, part six of C-Session 6 is wrap up and follows the protocol outlined in Sect. 8.4.7.1.

10.4 Step-by-Step Guidelines to Implement C-Session 7

C-Session 7 builds on C-Session 6 and focuses on helping children manage their fears by climbing Bravery Ladders.

As usual, prior to the start of the group, the child group therapists discuss the roles each will play in the session. At the appropriate start time, at least two child and/or parent group therapists greet parents and children in the waiting room and direct them to the parent and child group rooms. As seen in Table 10.3, there are six parts to C-Session 7.

10.4.1 Part One of C-Session 7

Part one of C-Session 7 (Circle Time) takes five to ten minutes to complete and begins with the usual protocol of welcoming the children, distributing name tags, discussing events or activities children wish to share with others, asking children if they practiced Spaghetti Arms and Toes, Balloon Breathing, and Imagery (and providing stickers or other reinforcements for practicing), and practicing Spaghetti Arms and Toes, Balloon Breathing, and Imagery for a few minutes (dimming the lights, if feasible; the child group therapists ensure that the children use the correct techniques, providing support and direction as needed).

The child group therapist taking the lead for this part of the session then:

1. Asks the children to name the three Tricks that Sneaky Fears play (Not Telling the Truth, Exaggerating, and Only Showing the Bad Things) and the three Trick Stoppers (Ignore Sneaky Fears, Think Brave Thoughts, and Talk to an Adult), while encouraging the children to call out the various Tricks and Trick Stoppers

Table 10.3 Outline of C-Session 7 (excerpt from Table 6.4)

Session[a]	Child group	
	Minutes	
7	5–10	Circle Time—review of events that might have happened to the children since the last session, topics covered in the previous session, and relaxation strategies
	10	Story Time—Chap. 7 of the children's story[b] and discussion of story
	15	How to Climb Bravery Ladders
	10	Craft Time
	5	Snack Time
	<1	Wrap up

[a]45- to 50-minute session; [b]Children's story section of *Taming Sneaky Fears—Leo the Lion's story of bravery & Inside Leo's den: The workbook* (Benoit & Monga, 2018a, b); <: less than

and writing these down on the white board (or flip chart) as the review takes place.

2. Encourages the children to share examples of what Tricks their own Sneaky Fears have played on their brain since the last session and what Trick Stoppers they used to start taming their Sneaky Fears.

Before distributing the puppets, the children are asked if they know how many more times they will be meeting as a group. Usually, at least one of the children is able to indicate that only two group sessions remain. The lead child group therapist ensures that the children are aware that only two group sessions remain after today's session.

The puppets are then distributed and each child chooses a puppet to hold for the next part of C-Session 7.

10.4.2   Part Two of C-Session 7

As seen in Table 10.3, part two of C-Session 7 (Story Time and discussion of story) takes about ten minutes to complete. The child group therapist taking the lead for reading the story reads Story Chap. 7 of *Taming Sneaky Fears—Leo the Lion's story of bravery & Inside Leo's den: The workbook* (Benoit & Monga, 2018a, b) with a lively and engaging voice and animated facial expressions while showing the illustrations. As in previous C-Sessions, one of the child group therapists plays the role of Sneaky Fears, saying Sneaky Fears' words in the story with a snarling and growling (or somewhat scary) voice.

10.4.2.1   Story Discussion

After Story Chap. 7 is read, the child group therapist leading the story discussion (three to four minutes in duration) asks:

1. If the children liked the story.
2. What Leo did in the story (Leo decided to build a Bravery Ladder with his mother so that he could speak to his teacher at school).

Before moving on to part three, the puppets are returned to the puppet container.

10.4.3   Part Three of C-Session 7

As seen in Table 10.3, part three of C-Session 7 (How to Climb Bravery Ladders) takes about ten minutes to complete. The child group therapist leading this portion of the session:

1. Asks the children if they have been climbing their Bravery Ladders.
2. Reviews the relevant version of the Bravery Ladder for Being Friendly with the children by asking them to place the correct Velcro illustrations on the correct steps (as described in Sections "Groups of Children Who Have Various Fears" and "Groups of Children with Selective Mutism and/or Social Anxiety Disorder").
3. Asks the children to show where they are on the Bravery Ladder by asking each (or at least some volunteers) to point to the ladder step they are on (more relevant for groups with children with selective mutism and/or social anxiety who are working on increasing the volume of their voice).
4. Reminds the children that Leo had to be really patient when he was climbing his Bravery Ladder because his Sneaky Fears were so used to being the boss of Leo's body and brain that they had little tantrums when Leo tried to Climb his Bravery Ladder, and so the children also have to be patient when climbing their own Bravery Ladders because their own Sneaky Fears are likely to put up a fuss when the children try to Climb their own Bravery Ladder.
5. Reminds the children that although Leo felt really scared and nervous while climbing his Bravery Ladder, he used Spaghetti Arms and Toes, Balloon Breathing, and Imagery to get his Feeling Thermometer down so that he was the Boss of his Body.
6. Reminds the children how Leo used his Trick Stoppers to Be the Boss of his Brain and how he was able to climb small steps on his Bravery Ladder for speaking at school with his teacher.
7. Emphasizes that when Leo climbed a few steps on his Bravery Ladder, Leo's Sneaky Fears became tamed as they became little jackal puppies and were no longer scary jackals.

10.4.4   Part Four of C-Session 7

As seen in Table 10.3, part four of C-Session 7 (Craft Time) takes about ten minutes to complete and follows the general protocol outlined in Sect. 8.4.5.1. One of the child group therapists leads the craft activity by explaining what is required and demonstrating what to draw on the white board (or flip chart) as needed. The other child group therapists distribute the Supplementary Child Workbook, ensure that the children are on the correct page, and go from child to child to provide support and direction as needed. Craft Time for C-Session 7 consists of only one drawing.

The drawing for C-Session 7 is found on page 5 of the Supplementary Child Workbook. The lead child group therapist completes the following tasks:

1. Draws a Bravery Ladder on the white board (or flip chart) with two boxes (similar to the illustration on page 5 of the Supplementary Child Workbook).
2. Reminds the children that when they are at the bottom of their Bravery Ladder their Sneaky Fears are wild and annoying.

3. Asks the children to draw a picture of what Sneaky Fears look like when Sneaky Fears are the boss of their (the children's) body and brain and the children are at the bottom of their Bravery Ladder.
4. Draws, as needed, a picture of the jackal-like Sneaky Fears looking wild and playing Tricks on the children in the bottom box on the white board (or flip chart).
5. Reminds the children that when they have climbed to the top of their Bravery Ladder and are brave, they will have tamed their Sneaky Fears.
6. Asks the children to draw a picture of what their Sneaky Fears will look like when their Sneaky Fears are all tame and the children have reached the top of their Bravery Ladder and are brave.
7. Draws, as needed, a picture of the jackal-like Sneaky Fears with leashes on them looking all tamed in the top box on the white board (or flip chart).

10.4.5   Part Five of C-Session 7

As seen in Table 10.3, part five of C-Session 7 is Snack Time and follows the protocol outlined in Sect. 8.4.6.1. The child group therapists gather information from each child during Snack Time about what they like to do so that some personalized details can be added to each Graduation Certificate as further discussed in Chap. 11.

10.4.6   Part Six of C-Session 7

As seen in Table 10.3, part six of C-Session 7 is wrap up and follows the protocol outlined in Sect. 8.4.7.1.

References

Benoit, D., & Monga, S. (2018a). *Apprivoiser les Peurs-pas-fines—L'histoire de bravoure de Léo le lionceau & Dans la tanière de Léo: Le cahier de travail*. Victoria, British Columbia: FriesenPress.
Benoit, D., & Monga, S. (2018b). *Taming Sneaky Fears: Leo the Lion's story of bravery & Inside Leo's den: The workbook*. Victoria, British Columbia: FriesenPress.
Huebner, D. (2006). *What to do when you worry too much—A kid's guide to overcoming anxiety*. Washington, DC: Magination Press.
Manassis, K. (2008). *Keys to parenting your anxious child* (2nd ed.). Hauppauge, NY: Barron's Educational Series.

Chapter 11
The Taming Sneaky Fears Program:
The Pivotal Role of Parents

11.1 Overview and Rationale

In the Taming Sneaky Fears program, a strong emphasis is placed on the essential role that parents play in helping their young children master the various concepts, strategies, and skills the children learn during their group sessions. Without the parents' active involvement in implementing the Taming Sneaky Fears program outside of sessions and in getting their young children to regularly practice the various strategies learned during group sessions, it is unlikely that the children would overcome their fears, learn to effectively manage their incapacitating anxiety symptoms, and benefit from the Taming Sneaky Fears program as much as hoped.

The Introduction Session and P-Sessions 1–3 equip parents with the necessary knowledge about CBT concepts, terminology, and strategies to help their four- to seven-year-old anxious children manage their anxiety symptoms. In P-Session 4, parents learn to manage oppositional, defiant, and non-compliant behaviors in their young anxious children, using the 1-2-3 Magic method. As P-Session 4 represents the mid-point in the Taming Sneaky Fears program, a brief feedback meeting with parents and child group therapists takes place immediately after P-Session 4 or just prior to P-Session 5. In P Session 5, parents learn to manage problem behavior around bedtime and nighttime, which are common problems in young anxious children. Parents also learn the importance of humor (and if time allows, parent group therapists review materials covered so far). During P-Sessions 6 and 7 and the first part of P-Session 8, the parent group therapists review concepts and strategies parents learned during the Taming Sneaky Fears program, focusing on concepts parents might be struggling with and issues that are relevant to the specific children in the group (for example, if a majority of children are socially anxious and selectively mute, most of the time will likely be spent on reviewing and refining Bravery Ladders parents

© Springer Nature Switzerland AG 2018
S. Monga and D. Benoit, *Assessing and Treating Anxiety Disorders in Young Children*, https://doi.org/10.1007/978-3-030-04939-3_11

have developed). Typically, a large portion of these review sessions focuses on the development of Bravery Ladders and problem solving around difficulties encountered during implementation of Bravery Ladders, as Bravery Ladders help conquer not only fear of social interactions and fear of being seen and heard speaking, but numerous other fears such as fear of being away from parental figures, fear of making mistakes (perfectionism), fear of animals, etc. Parents are encouraged to play an active role in providing feedback to other parents and helping to problem solve difficulties discussed during these parent sessions.

For the last 15 minutes of P-Session 8 (and C-Session 8), the children and parents and all the child and parent group therapists meet together in the parent group room for a brief graduation ceremony, which consists of handing out to each child a graduation certificate (Fig. 11.1) and the two workbooks each child used during the sessions, i.e., *Taming Sneaky Fears—Leo the Lion's story of bravery & Inside Leo's den: The workbook* (Benoit & Monga, 2018a, b) and the Supplementary Child Workbook[1] that contains the additional drawings the children completed as part of Craft Time at each session. During the graduation portion of P- and C-Session 8, the lead child group therapist reminds parents and children of the various strategies the children have learned to tame their Sneaky Fears and be brave. The lead child group therapist also reminds children (and parents) that, just like Leo the Lion and Ellie the Elephant did in the story, they need to continue to use and practice their strategies in order to keep their tamed Sneaky Fears from becoming wild again.

Fig. 11.1 Example of a graduation certificate

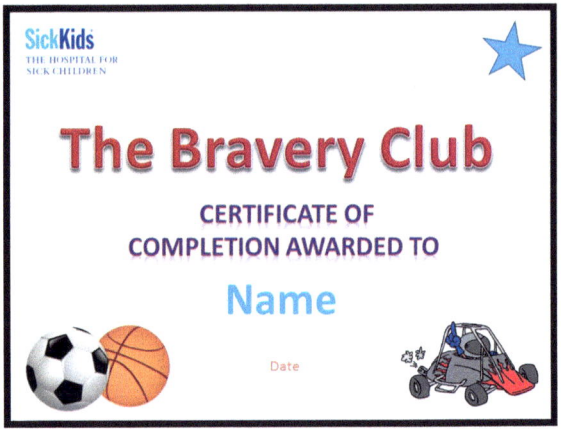

11.2 Step-by-Step Guidelines to Implement the Parent Feedback Meeting[2]

As seen in Table 11.1, immediately after P-Session 4 ends, the child group thera-pists meet with each of the children's parent(s), one child's parent(s) at a time, for approximately 5 minutes to hear a brief summary of how the child is doing outside of the group and to provide each parent with a brief summary of how the child is engaging and doing in the group sessions with peers and child group therapists. The child group therapists divide the task of meeting with the parents among themselves and use the schedule of five-minute appointment times that was completed by the parents during P-Session 3 (as described in Sect. 10.2.1).

The meeting with each child's parent(s) takes place without the child (if two child group therapists provide the Taming Sneaky Fears group program, one of the child group therapists stays with the child in the waiting area or in a separate room while the other child group therapist meets with the child's parent(s); if more than two child group therapists are involved in delivering the Taming Sneaky Fears program, one of the child group therapists stays with the children while the other two child group therapists divide among themselves the appointment times with the parents.

When in a separate room with each child's parent(s), the child group therapist:

1. Informs the parent(s) that it is hard to believe that we are already half way through the group program and that today is an opportunity for parents to provide a brief summary, whether it is positive or not so positive, of how their child is doing outside of group, and also an opportunity for them to hear about how their child is doing in the group.
2. Invites the parent(s) to specifically provide a brief summary of any changes (whether they are positive or not so positive) the parent(s) noted in the child since the start of the group program.
3. Is mindful not to engage in discussion about implementation of strategies with the parent(s) (as this is a focus of the parent group sessions) and keeps the discussion focused on how each child is progressing and continues to refocus the parent(s) on the changes the parent(s) noted in the child.
4. Provides a brief summary of how the child is engaging with peers and child group therapists and whether the child appears to understand the group program concepts, for example, by commenting on whether the child is paying attention and listening to the story, participating in the discussion verbally or non-verbally, and completing the drawing(s) and/or socializing with peers.
5. Asks whether the parent(s) practice(s) strategies with the child (if and when the parent(s) report(s) no improvement in the child's symptoms or functioning).
6. Informs the parent(s) that by the end of C-Session 5, the children will have learned all of the main strategies and that going forward practice of all the strategies and

---

[2]The Parent Feedback meeting occurs immediately after P-Session 4 or immediately before the Start of P-Session 5

skills discussed during sessions is essential for the children to fully benefit from the Taming Sneaky Fears program.

7. Informs the parent(s) that in C-Sessions 6 and 7, the children will learn How to Climb Bravery Ladders and as such, each child will likely be eager to climb his or her own Bravery Ladders.

Typically, a maximum of 5 minutes is allocated to meet with each child's parent(s) to ensure that all the parents meet with a child group therapist after P-Session 4 ends (and as needed, immediately prior to the start of P-Session 5). After all the appointments have taken place, all child and parent group therapists meet to discuss the feedback parents provided with respect to the children's progress outside of sessions.

11.3   Step-by-Step Guidelines to Implement P-Session 4

Prior to the start of P-Session 4, the parent group therapists determine which therapists are in charge of each specific part of P-Session 4 and ensure that all the materials needed (as listed in Table 6.3) are available in the parent group room, and specifically, that the 1-2-3 Magic DVD and equipment to view it are available.

As P-Session 4 is about to start, at least two child and/or parent group therapists go to the waiting area to greet all parents and children and bring them to their respective room.[3]

As seen in Table 11.1, P-Session 4 in the Taming Sneaky Fears program is divided into three main parts.

Table 11.1   Outline of P-Session 4 (excerpt from Table 6.4)

Session[a]	Parent group	
	Minutes	
4	5	Overview of the 1-2-3 Magic program
	45	Watch the 1-2-3 Magic video
	<1	Wrap up
	*Child group therapists meet with each child's parent(s) for five minutes **at the end of Session 4** and (as needed) **immediately prior to the beginning of Session 5** to provide and receive feedback on each child's progress*	

[a]45- to 50-minute session; <: less than

---

[3]If parents are in charge of bringing the snacks for the child group sessions, it is typically at that moment that the parent who brings the snack gives it to one of the child group therapists.

11.3.1 Part One of P-Session 4

As occurs with each parent session, one of the parent group therapists welcomes the parents and invites them to take their name tag from the table and put it on as they make themselves comfortable. If parents are in charge of bringing in the snack for the children, the lead parent group therapist reminds the parents of who is in charge of bringing in the snack for the next session. The parent group therapists also remind parents of their scheduled appointments for the feedback session with the child group therapists from the list completed during P-Session 3.

Part one of P-Session 4 (overview of the 1-2-3 Magic) takes two or three minutes to complete. It is brief to allow parents to view as much of the 1-2-3 Magic DVD as possible during the session. The parent group therapist who takes the lead for this part:

1. Shows the parents the 1-2-3 Magic DVD, More 1-2-3 Magic DVD, and 1-2-3 Magic book, indicating to parents that the entire session today focuses on watching as much of the 1-2-3 Magic DVD as time allows, to help parents manage more effectively the oppositional and non-compliant behavior often displayed by young anxious children; therefore, there will not be time for a question period today, but all the upcoming sessions will include enough time for questions.
2. States that the areas discussed today correspond to item 12 (Use the 1-2-3 Magic) of the What to Do to Help list (Fig. 4 of the Parent Manual).
3. Mentions to the parents that time will allow the viewing of only a portion of the DVD during today's session.
4. Instructs the parents to read on their own the text provided in the Parent Manual for Session 4 (and points out the page number where parents can find this information).
5. Asks the parents to start implementing the 1-2-3 Magic method at home as this is a new task as seen in the Parent Session 4 Tasks of the Parent Manual.

11.3.2 Part Two of P-Session 4

Part two of P-Session 4 takes approximately 45 minutes to complete and consists of viewing as much of the 1-2-3 Magic DVD as time allows.

11.3.3 Part Three of P-Session 4

Part three of P-Session 4 (wrap up) takes 30–60 seconds to complete and as mentioned in the protocols of previous P-Sessions, it starts when one of the child group therapists knocks at the door and enters the parent group room to provide a ten-second summary of the topic covered during the child session that day. As soon as the child group therapist departs, the lead parent group therapist thanks parents for their attention and cooperation during today's session, and reminds:

1. All parents to:

    a. Remove their name tags and place them on the table as these are re-used at each session.
    b. Go to the children's group room to pick up their children.

2. The parents who are meeting with the child group therapists at the end of today's Session 4 to wait with their child in the waiting area and the child group therapists will meet them in the waiting area at the pre-arranged time.

3. The parents who are meeting with the child group therapists just before the start of the next session (Session 5) to come early to register for the clinic and meet the child group therapists at the pre-arranged time (the child group therapists will meet them in the waiting area at the pre-arranged time).

11.4   Step-by-Step Guidelines to Implement P-Session 5

As described in Sect. 11.2, and as seen in Table 11.2, immediately prior to the beginning of P-Session 5, the child group therapists continue to meet individually with whichever parent(s) they were not able to meet at the end of Session 4.

Prior to the start of P-Session 5, the parent group therapists determine which therapists are in charge of each specific part of P-Session 5 and ensure that all the materials needed (as listed in Table 6.3) are available in the parent group room.

Table 11.2 Outline of P-Session 5 (excerpt from Table 6.4)

Session[a]	Parent group	
	Minutes	
5	*Child group therapists meet with each child's parent(s) for five minutes **at the end of Session 4** and (as needed) **immediately prior to the beginning of Session 5** to provide and receive feedback on each child's progress*	
	5–10	Brave moments and effective praise
	5–10	Review of other tasks
	30–40	Common problem: Sleep; importance of humor; review of Bravery Ladders
	<1	Wrap up

[a]45- to 50-minute session; <: less than

As P-Session 5 is about to start, at least two child and/or parent group therapists go to the waiting area to greet all parents and children and bring them to their respective room.[4]

As seen in Table 11.2, P-Session 5 in the Taming Sneaky Fears program is divided into four main parts.

11.4.1   Part One of P-Session 5

As occurs with each parent session, one of the parent group therapists welcomes the parents and invites them to take their name tag from the table and put it on as they make themselves comfortable. If parents are in charge of bringing in the snack for the children, the lead parent group therapist thanks the parent(s) who brought the snack for today's session and reminds the parents of who is in charge of bringing in the snack for the next session.

As seen in Table 11.2, part one of P-Session 5 (brave moments and effective praise) takes five to ten minutes to complete. As done in previous P-Sessions, the parent group therapist leading this part of P-Session 5 asks two or three parents to volunteer examples of brave moments they noticed in their children since the previous session and how they provided effective praise. The lead parent group therapist then follows the same protocol used in previous sessions:

1. Invites supportive comments from other parents on what the parents volunteering examples did well when providing effective praise and what they could have done differently to provide even more effective praise.
2. Asks the parents to review the three main characteristics of effective praise (i.e., start praise with a '*You*' statement, focus on the *specific behavior* displayed by the child, provide praise *as soon as possible* after the display of the brave behavior).
3. Asks the parents to review the rationale for identifying brave moments and providing effective praise (i.e., the more one pays attention to a behavior, the more likely the behavior is to be repeated).
4. Reminds the parents that focusing on brave moments and providing effective praise are tasks to do throughout the program as outline in the Parent Session 5 Tasks of the Parent Manual (and ideally, would continue even after the Taming Sneaky Fears program is completed).

Throughout this part, the lead parent therapist actively provides constructive feedback to the parents who volunteer examples and comments.

---

[4]If parents are in charge of bringing the snacks for the child group sessions, it is typically at that moment that the parent who brings the snack gives it to one of the child group therapists.

11.4.2   Part Two of P-Session 5

As seen in Table 11.2, part two of P-Session 5 (review of other tasks) takes 5–10 minutes to complete. The parent group therapist leading this part:

1. Asks the parents to volunteer how they implemented the various tasks outlined in P-Session 4, i.e., help their children be Feeling Catchers, use Body Scans, and do the various relaxation strategies; start to develop a Bravery Ladder (but not implement it yet as the children learn about Bravery Ladders only in their Sessions 6 and 7); and use strategies for managing excessive worries.
2. Asks who has implemented the 1-2-3 Magic approach.
3. Encourages the parents to share their successes and struggles in implementing 1-2-3 Magic and share ideas with other parents about how to implement 1-2-3 Magic successfully.
4. Reminds the parents of the two rules to follow when implementing 1-2-3 Magic, i.e., *No Talking* and *No Emotion*.
5. Reminds the parents that these aforementioned tasks continue to be tasks we recommend parents use consistently in between sessions (and points out the page number in the Parent Manual[5] listing these and the specific tasks to do after today's session).

11.4.3   Part Three of P-Session 5

Part three of P-Session 5 takes 30–40 minutes to complete. It begins when the parent group therapist leading this part:

1. Asks the parents to go to Session 5 in their Parent Manual (and points out the page number where the information is located).
2. Mentions to the parents that today in the children's group, the children learn about the Feeling Thermometer, so starting today, parents could use the Feeling Thermometer (information provided in P-Session 1 and Fig. 8 of the Parent Manual) to help the children figure out the intensity of the feelings they experience.
3. Shows the parents the children's workbooks (the workbook section of *Taming Sneaky Fears—Leo the Lion's story of bravery & Inside Leo's den: The workbook* (Benoit & Monga, 2018a, b) and the Supplementary Child Workbook and what drawings the children do during their session, i.e., My Feeling Thermometer for nervous or scared and My Feeling Thermometer for shy.
4. Encourages the parents to ask their children to do a similar craft at home that shows not only examples of times when their child was nervous or scared (and then shy) at a 1 or 2 on the Feeling Thermometer, then at a 5 or 6, then at a 9 or 10, but also includes the Body Scan corresponding to the different intensities of

---

[5]The Parent Manual is provided as one of the Supplementary Materials in Chap. 6.

emotions, to show the child that their body feels different with different intensities of the same emotion, for example, when children feel nervous or scared

   a. At a 1 or 2 on the Feeling Thermometer, they can startle just a little—as in the example of her cousin Eleanor the Elephant jumping out from behind a couch that Ellie the Elephant provides in the story.

   b. At a 5 or 6 on the Feeling Thermometer, they can feel their heart beating fast and have butterflies in their tummy.

   c. At a 9 or 10 on the Feeling Thermometer, their heart can beat hard and fast, they can find it hard to breathe, they could feel like their tummy is sore and they are about to throw up, they could sweat and shake, their throat could feel tight, their voice could be stuck in their throat, etc.

5. Indicates that in the parents' Session 5 today, we focus on two main points: (1) a common problem seen in young anxious children (sleep—difficulty with settling at bedtime and nighttime waking) and (2) the usefulness of humor in helping young children manage anxiety symptoms.
6. Mentions that if time allows, we will also review one or more Bravery Ladders parents have developed for their children.
7. Proceeds with covering the psychoeducation topics for today's Session 5 (as described above), using the Parent Manual as basis to deliver part three of P-Session 5.

11.4.3.1 Common Problem—Sleep

The parent group therapist leading this part:

1. Asks the parents to go to the relevant section of the Parent Manual and points out the page number where this information is located in the Parent Manual.
2. Asks the parents to indicate (with a show of hands) who has a child with a sleep problem, i.e., trouble falling asleep, trouble staying asleep, or trouble sleeping alone without the parent(s) being present (the parent group therapist emphasizes that the question is about children who are participating in the group, not their siblings):

   a. If there are no children with sleep problems, then the lead parent group therapist does not go over the information on bedtime and nighttime waking from the Parent Manual, and instead only points out that should the children ever develop difficulties with falling asleep or staying asleep, we suggest (1) following Dr. Phelan's recommendations to manage sleep problems, as summarized in their Parent Manual; and (2) reading the section of Dr. Phelan's book that deals with bedtime behavior and nighttime waking; the lead parent group therapist then goes on to the next topic of P-Session 5 (humor).

   b. If at least one child in the group has trouble settling to sleep or staying asleep, then the lead parent group therapist:

    i. Emphasizes that most of the information on the topic of how to manage sleep difficulties that is covered during today's Session 5 is a summary from Dr. Phelan's 1-2-3 Magic book so parents are encouraged to read Dr. Phelan's book chapters on bedtime behavior and nighttime waking.

    ii. Mentions that the suggestions in the Parent Manual are meant for parents who wish for their young children to learn to fall asleep on their own, stay in bed at bedtime, and stay in their own bed through the night; they are not meant for parents who choose to co-sleep and value co-sleeping for a variety of cultural or other reasons.

    iii. Goes over the Basic Bedtime Method as described in the Parent Manual, asking the parents to follow along and pointing out the page number where this information is located in the Parent Manual.

    iv. Indicates that as mentioned by Dr. Phelan in his book (and summarized in the Parent Manual), many children will respond immediately to the Basic Bedtime Method, but other children will not comply so readily.

    v. Points out to the parents the section in the Parent Manual where information about "some problems that might come up" and invites parents to read that section more thoroughly at home if they consider using the Basic Bedtime Method as we are not going to go over this section in detail during today's session.

    vi. Reviews the Nighttime Waking and Scary Dreams sections as described in the Parent Manual, asking the parents to follow along and pointing out the page number where this information is located in the Parent Manual.

3. Uses Fig. 4 in the Parent Manual to point out that as seen in item 13 of the What to Do to Help list, we encourage parents of young anxious children to use a sleep program as needed.

4. Reminds the parents that a new task to do after today's session (for parents who have children with sleep problems) is to implement a sleep program, in addition to the other tasks previously mentioned tasks (and points out the page number in the Parent Manual listing Parent Session 5 Tasks).

11.4.3.2   Humor

The parent group therapist leading this part:

1. Reviews the relevant section of the Parent Manual and points out the page number where this information is located.

2. Emphasizes that humor:

    a. Helps children manage their anxiety symptoms.

    b. Involves a capacity to place one's behavior into perspective and think of a situation in a new and fresh way, in a way that makes children laugh and relax.

   c. Helps children to realize that when they are having fun and laughing, they do not feel shy or nervous or scared, so humor can be like a Trick Stopper and can help to tame Sneaky Fears.

3. Uses Fig. 4 to point out that as seen in item 11 of the What to Do to Help list, we encourage parents of young anxious children to use humor and help them learn the difference between humor and self-deprecation and making fun of others.
4. Reminds the parents that another new task for after today's session is to use humor (and points out the page number in the Parent Manual listing Parent Session 5 Tasks).

11.4.3.3 Review of Bravery Ladders

If time allows, the parent group therapist leading this part:

1. Asks the parents for volunteers to present the Bravery Ladders they have developed for their children; this represents an opportunity for parent group therapists to help parents review the various principles discussed in P-Session 3.
2. Reminds the parents not to start using Bravery Ladders yet, as the children will be introduced to the concept of Climbing Bravery Ladders only at the next two sessions (Sessions 6 and 7).

11.4.4 Part Four of P-Session 5

As seen in Table 11.2, part four of P-Session 5 (wrap up) takes 30–60 seconds to complete. As mentioned in the protocols of previous P-Sessions, it starts when one of the child group therapists knocks at the door and enters the parent group room to provide a ten-second summary of the topics covered during the child session that day. As done in all previous sessions, as soon as the child group therapist departs, the lead parent therapist thanks parents for their attention and cooperation during today's session, and reminds parents:

1. That the child group therapist coming in is the signal for the parent group session to end promptly as the children are ready to be picked up.
2. To remove their name tags and place them on the table as these are re-used at each session.
3. To go to the children's group room to pick up their children.

11.5   Step-by-Step Guidelines to Implement P-Sessions 6 and 7

Prior to the start of P-Sessions 6 and 7, the parent group therapists determine which therapists are in charge of each specific part of P-Sessions 6 and 7 and ensure that all the materials needed (as listed in Table 6.3) are available in the parent group room.

As previously done for each session, when each of P-Session 6 and P-Session 7 is about to start, at least two child and/or parent group therapists go to the waiting area to greet all parents and children and bring them to their respective room.[6]

At the beginning of each of P-Session 6 and P-Session 7, the lead parent group therapist mentions how many sessions are left in the program, what topics the children are covering in their own session that day, and what drawings they will do:

1. For C-Session 6, the children learn How to Climb My Bravery Ladder to overcome fears; the parent group therapist shows the parents page 80 of *Taming Sneaky Fears—Leo the Lion's story of bravery & Inside Leo's den: The workbook* (Benoit & Monga, 2018a, b), which the children will use to draw a picture of "Me at the Bottom of My Bravery Ladder" (i.e., nervous and scared or shy) and 'Me at the Top of My Bravery Ladder' (i.e., brave).
2. For C-Session 7, the children continue to work on the concept of climbing Bravery Ladders to overcome fears and review all the concepts they have learned in the group to date; their drawing is a picture of 'My Sneaky Fears at the Bottom of my Bravery Ladder' (i.e., all wild and bossy) and 'My Sneaky Fears at the Top of My Bravery Ladder' (i.e., all tame); the lead parent group therapist shows the parents page 5 of the Supplementary Child Workbook, which the children will use for their drawing.

In P-Session 7, the lead parent group therapist reminds the parents that Session 8 is the last session of the Taming Sneaky Fears program and is abbreviated (lasts approximately 40 minutes instead of the usual 45–50 minutes with the last 15 minutes consisting of a brief graduation for the children after the children come to the parent group room).

As seen in Table 11.3, P-Sessions 6 and 7 in the Taming Sneaky Fears program are divided into four parts.

11.5.1   Part One of P-Sessions 6 and 7

As occurs with each parent session, one of the parent group therapists welcomes the parents and invites them to take their name tag from the table and put it on as they make themselves comfortable. If parents are in charge of bringing in the snack for the children, the lead parent group therapist thanks the parent(s) who brought the

---

[6]If parents are in charge of bringing the snacks for the child group sessions, it is typically at that moment that the parent who brings the snack gives it to one of the child group therapists.

Table 11.3 Outline of P-Sessions 6 and 7 (excerpt from Table 6.4)

Sessions[a]	Parent group	
	Minutes	
6 and 7	5–10	Brave moments and effective praise
	5–10	Review of other tasks
	30–40	Review of all materials covered to date
	<1	Wrap up

[a]45- to 50-minute session
<:less than

snack and in P-Session-6 reminds the parents of who is in charge of bringing in the snack for P-Session 7 (there is no snack provided at Session 8).

As seen in Table 11.3, part one of P-Sessions 6 and 7 (brave moments and effective praise) takes 5–10 minutes to complete. As done in previous P-Sessions, the parent group therapist leading this part of P-Sessions 6 and 7 asks two or three parents to volunteer examples of brave moments they noticed in their children since the previous session and how they provided effective praise. As usual, the lead parent group therapist:

1. Invites supportive comments from other parents on what the parents volunteering examples did well when providing effective praise and what they could have done differently to provide even more effective praise.
2. Asks the parents to review the three main characteristics of effective praise (i.e., start praise with a '*You*' statement, focus on the *specific behavior* displayed by the child, provide praise *as soon as possible* after the display of the brave behavior).
3. Asks the parents to review the rationale for identifying brave moments and providing effective praise (i.e., the more one pays attention to a behavior, the more likely the behavior is to be repeated).
4. Reminds the parents that focusing on brave moments and providing effective praise are tasks to do in-between sessions throughout the program (and ideally, would continue even after the Taming Sneaky Fears program is completed).

Throughout this part, the lead parent therapist actively provides constructive feedback to the parents who volunteer examples and comments.

11.5.2   Part Two of P-Sessions 6 and 7

As seen in Table 11.3, part two of P-Sessions 6 and 7 (review of other tasks) takes 5–10 minutes to complete. The parent group therapist leading this part:

1. Asks the parents to volunteer how they implemented the various tasks outlined in previous parent sessions (i.e., help their children be Feeling Catchers, use Body Scans, and do the various relaxation strategies; be Trick Catchers and use the Stop

sign and the Trick Stoppers; start to develop a Bravery Ladder (but not implement it yet as the children learn about Bravery Ladders only in their Sessions 6 and 7); use strategies for managing excessive worries; use Dr. Phelan's 1-2-3 Magic program; use a sleep program as needed; and use humor.

2. Reminds the parents that these aforementioned tasks are tasks we recommend parents do between sessions throughout the program (and points out the page numbers in the Parent Manual where Parent Session 6 Tasks (after P-Session 6) and Parent Session 7 Tasks (after P-Session 7) are located.

11.5.3   Part Three of P-Sessions 6 and 7

Part three of P-Sessions 6 and 7 each takes 30–40 minutes to complete. It begins when the parent group therapist leading this part:

1. Reminds the parents of how many sessions are left before the conclusion of the Taming Sneaky Fears program.
2. Mentions to the parents that in their Sessions 6 and 7, the children learn about How to Climb Bravery Ladders, so starting today, parents could use the language of Climbing a Bravery Ladder.
3. Shows the parents what drawings the children do during their Sessions 6 and 7, using the children's workbooks (*Taming Sneaky Fears—Leo the Lion's story of bravery & Inside Leo's den: The workbook* (Benoit & Monga, 2018a, b) and the Supplementary Child Workbook.
4. Indicates that in the parents' Sessions 6 and 7, we focus on reviewing all the concepts discussed in the program to date.
5. Asks for volunteers to present the Bravery Ladders parents have been working on.
6. Invites the other parents to discuss what aspects of the Bravery Ladders are likely to work well (and why) and what aspects of the Bravery Ladders might need improvement (and why and how to improve).
7. Is careful not to take over, but instead lets the parents take an increasingly greater role in coming up with solutions and suggestions, and in constructively critiquing the work they and other parents do.
8. Might focus more on how to manage excessive worries than Bravery Ladders (or any other topic covered during the program to date, depending on the needs of each group).

11.5.4   Part Four of P-Sessions 6 and 7

As seen in Table 11.3, part four of P-Sessions 6 and 7 (wrap up) takes 30–60 seconds to complete. As mentioned in the protocols of previous P-Sessions, it starts when one of the child group therapists knocks at the door and enters the parent group room to provide a ten-second summary of the topic covered during the child session that day. As soon as the child group therapist departs, the lead parent therapist thanks parents for their attention and cooperation during today's session, and reminds parents:

1. That the child group therapist coming in is the signal for the parent group session to end promptly as the children are ready to be picked up.
2. To remove their name tags and place them on the table as these are re-used at each session.
3. To go to the children's group room to pick up their children.

11.6   Step-by-Step Guidelines to Implement P-Session 8

Session 8 is the last session of the Taming Sneaky Fears program.

As usual, prior to the start of P-Session 8, the parent group therapists determine which therapists are in charge of each specific part of P-Session 8 and ensure that all the materials needed (as listed in Table 6.3) are available in the parent group room.

As previously done for each session, when P-Session 8 is about to start, at least two child and/or parent group therapists go to the waiting area to greet all parents and children and bring them to their respective room. As seen in Table 11.4, there are only two parts to P-Session 8.

Table 11.4 Outline of P- Session 8 and C-Session 8 (excerpt from Table 6.4)

Session[a]	Parent group		Child group	
	Minutes		Minutes	
8	5–25	Review	5	Circle Time—review of events that might have happened to the children since the last session, topics covered in the previous sessions, and relaxation
			10	Story Time—Chapter 8 of children's story[b] and discussion of story
			10	Review of all concepts
	15	Children come in for graduation	15	Children go to parent group room for graduation

[a]40-minute session; children and parent groups run concurrently, but in separate rooms for the first 25 minutes then the children come to the parents' room for graduation
[b]Children's story section of *Taming Sneaky Fears—Leo the Lion's story of bravery & Inside Leo's den: The workbook* (Benoit & Monga, 2018a, b)

11.6.1   Part One of P-Session 8

At the beginning of P-Session 8, the parent group therapist who takes the lead for this part:

1. Mentions that today is the last session of the Taming Sneaky Fears program.
2. Indicates what topics the children are covering in their own session that day, i.e., the children review all the concepts they have learned during the program.
3. Shows the parents page 88 of one of the children's workbooks, *Taming Sneaky Fears—Leo the Lion's story of bravery & Inside Leo's den: The workbook* (Benoit & Monga, 2018a, b), and indicates that during today's session, the children draw a picture of 'My Tamed Sneaky Fears.'
4. Reminds the parents that the children will come to the parent group room for the last 15 minutes or so of today's Session 8 for 'graduation' where they will be given a certificate and the two workbooks they used during the sessions (*Taming Sneaky Fears—Leo the Lion's story of bravery & Inside Leo's den: The workbook* (Benoit & Monga, 2018a, b) and the Supplementary Child Workbook) to take home.
5. Informs the parents that, as was mentioned in previous sessions, the workbook section of *Taming Sneaky Fears—Leo the Lion's story of bravery & Inside Leo's den: The workbook* (Benoit & Monga, 2018a, b) contains more drawings than the children could complete in the sessions, and encourages parents to have their children complete these drawings over the coming weeks in order to ensure that the materials and information from the group program are consolidated.
6. If relevant, discusses any follow-up plan, emphasizing that at this point, they, as parents, and their children, have all the tools needed to overcome the children's fears and worries, and what is needed is for them and their children to continue to practice all the strategies regularly until their children's own Sneaky Fears are tame (and, as needed, to continue to involve other adults, such as school personnel (for more details see Chap. 12), to implement Bravery Ladders and help to tame Sneaky Fears).
7. Points out that it might take considerably longer than the eight weeks of the program for the children to master all the strategies to tame their Sneaky Fears, and just like Leo the Lion did in the story, the children need to continue to work hard to tame their Sneaky Fears.
8. Mentions that it is usually recommended that parents and children practice and implement what they have learned during the program for at least three to four months before they seek additional follow up; most children and parents do not require additional follow up.
9. Invites the parents to ask any questions they might have.

11.6.2   Part Two of P-Session 8

Part two of P-Session 8 (graduation) begins when the children and child group therapists come to the parent group room and follows the protocol described in Sect. 11.7.4.

11.7   Step-by-Step Guidelines to Implement C-Session 8

Prior to the start of C-Session 8, the child group therapists determine which therapists are in charge of which specific part of C-Session 8 and ensure that all the materials needed (as listed in Table 6.3) are available in the child group room. In addition, the child group therapists prepare the certificates that will be handed out to the children during 'graduation' (Fig. 11.1). Each graduation certificate could have the name of the group (from C-Session 1), the name of the individual child, and if feasible, in order to further individualize each certificate, illustrations of a few things that each child specifically likes, which were obtained through discussions with the children during Snack Time in C-Sessions 6 and 7. The key concept in C-Session 8 is for the children to have a sense of accomplishment that they now have the skills to tame their Sneaky Fears and be brave.

As seen in Table 11.4, there are four parts to C-Session 8.

11.7.1   Part One of C-Session 8

Part one of C-Session 8 (Circle Time) takes five to ten minutes to complete and begins with the usual protocol of welcoming the children, distributing name tags, discussing events or activities children wish to share with others, asking children if they practiced Spaghetti Arms and Toes, Balloon Breathing, and Imagery (providing stickers or other reinforcements for practicing), and practicing Spaghetti Arms and Toes and Balloon Breathing for a few minutes, dimming the lights if feasible; the child group therapists ensure that the children use the correct techniques and provide support and direction as needed.

The child group therapist taking the lead for this portion of the session:

1. Asks the children if they have been climbing their Bravery Ladders.
2. Reviews the relevant Bravery Ladder (Bravery Ladder for Being Friendly or Bravery Ladder for Speaking to the Teacher at School) by asking the children to place the correct Velcro illustrations on the correct steps and asking children (or at least some volunteers) to show by pointing to the Ladder step they are on.
3. Asks the children to name the three Tricks that Sneaky Fears play (i.e., Not Telling the Truth, Exaggerating, and Only Showing the Bad Things) and the three Trick Stoppers (i.e., Ignore Sneaky Fears, Think Brave Thoughts, and Talk to an Adult), while encouraging the children to call out the various Tricks and Trick Stoppers and writing these down on the white board (or flip chart).
4. Encourages the children to share examples of what Tricks their own Sneaky Fears have played on their brain since the last session and what Trick Stoppers the children have used to start taming their Sneaky Fears.

The puppets are then distributed and each child chooses a puppet to hold during Part two of the session.

11.7.2 Part Two of C-Session 8

As seen in Table 11.4, part two of C-Session 8 (Story Time and discussion of story) takes about ten minutes to complete. The child group therapist taking the lead for reading the story reads Story Chap. 8 of *Taming Sneaky Fears—Leo the Lion's story of bravery & Inside Leo's den: The Workbook* (Benoit & Monga, 2018a, b), with a lively and engaging voice and animated facial expressions while showing the illustrations.

11.7.2.1 Story Discussion

After the story is read, the child group therapist leading the story discussion (three to four minutes in duration) asks:

1. If the children liked the story.
2. What Leo the Lion and Ellie the Elephant did in the story (Leo climbed all of the steps of his Bravery Ladder and was able to speak to his teacher; Ellie also climbed all of the steps of her Bravery Ladder so she was able to get to the top of her bunk bed; and both Ellie and Leo tamed their Sneaky Fears.

Before moving on to part three, the puppets are returned to the puppet container.

11.7.3 Part Three of C-Session 8

As seen in Table 11.4, part three of C-Session 8 (Craft Time) takes about ten minutes to complete and follows the general protocol outlined in Sect. 8.4.5.1. One of the child group therapists leads Craft Time by explaining what is required while the other child group therapists go from child to child to provide support and direction, as needed. The specific task for C-Session 8 is for each child to draw a picture of their tamed Sneaky Fears in the craft box found on page 88 of the workbook section of *Taming Sneaky Fears—Leo the Lion's story of bravery & Inside Leo's den: The workbook* (Benoit & Monga 2018a, b).

11.7.4 Part Four of C-Session 8

As seen in Table 11.4, part four of C-Session 8 is graduation and takes about 15 minutes to complete. For the graduation, the child group therapists escort the children to the parent group room and invite them to join their parents who are already seated in the parent group room. A short graduation ceremony then takes place. The child group therapist that leads the graduation ceremony:

1. Welcomes everyone.

2. Says a few words about how the group program has come to an end.
3. Calls the children, one by one, to the front of the room and gives them:

   a. A graduation certificate (Fig. 11.1) that includes the name of the group given by the children in C-Session 1, the name of the child, and, if possible, illustrations of activities (or characters, pets, etc.) that the child enjoys (details in Sects. 10.4.5 and 10.5.5).
   b. The two workbooks the children used to make their drawings during the sessions:
      i. *Taming Sneaky Fears—Leo the Lion's story of bravery & Inside Leo's den: The workbook* (Benoit & Monga, 2018a, b).
      ii. The Supplementary Child Workbook.

4. Invites all the parents, children, child group therapists, and parent group therapists to clap after each child receives the certificate and the workbooks.
5. Encourages the parents to spend a few minutes to review their child's workbooks with their child (after each child has come up to the front of the room to receive the graduation certificate and workbooks); parent and child group therapists can mingle with the parents and children during this time.
6. Thanks parents and children for attending and brings the group session to a conclusion after about five minutes of interactions between parents and their children.

References

Benoit, D., & Monga, S. (2018a). *Apprivoiser les Peurs-pas-fines—L'histoire de bravoure de Léo le lionceau & Dans la tanière de Léo: Le cahier de travail*. Victoria, British Columbia: FriesenPress.
Benoit, D., & Monga, S. (2018b). *Taming Sneaky Fears—Leo the Lion's story of bravery & Inside Leo's den: The workbook*. Victoria, British Columbia: FriesenPress.
Phelan, T. W. (2004a). *1-2-3 Magic DVD: Managing difficult behavior*. Glen Ellyn, IL: ParentMagic Inc.
Phelan, T. W. (2004b). *More 1-2-3 Magic DVD: Encouraging good behavior*. Glen Ellyn, IL: ParentMagic Inc.
Phelan, T. W. (2014). *1-2-3 Magic* (5th ed.). Glen Ellyn, IL: ParentMagic Inc.

Chapter 12
The Taming Sneaky Fears Program: Working with Daycare and School Professionals

12.1 Introduction[1]

Daycares and schools play a prominent role in the lives of many four- to seven-year-old anxious children. In fact, for some young anxious children, especially those with selective mutism, social anxiety, and separation anxiety, the implementation in the daycare or school setting of the strategies they learn in the Taming Sneaky Fears group Cognitive Behavior Therapy (CBT) program is often a necessary step to overcome their anxiety symptoms. Although, the full Taming Sneaky Fears group CBT program, or aspects of the program, could be implemented within a daycare or school setting by professionals working in these settings, the goals of this chapter are to:

1. Provide suggestions on how clinicians[2] can enable and support parents of four- to seven-year-old children with anxiety disorders to advocate for daycare and school supports.
2. Offer an approach to encourage daycare and school professionals and/or administrators[3] to implement evidence-based strategies from the Taming Sneaky Fears program in daycare or school settings.
3. Suggest what type of information and training clinicians might provide to daycare providers, teachers, and school administrators to equip them with the necessary knowledge and skills to help young anxious children and their parents implement

---

[1]This chapter uses several verbatim or slightly modified excerpts from chaps. 7–11 to bring together, in a distilled fashion, relevant information for clinicians and researchers to use in their work with daycare and school professionals to facilitate the implementation of Cognitive Behavior Therapy Strategies from the Taming Sneaky Fears Program in daycare and school settings

[2]From this point forward 'clinicians' refers to clinicians and, where relevant, researchers working with young anxious children and their parents.

[3]From this point forward, 'school administrators' refers to principals and other lead administrators in schools and school boards and administrators in daycare settings.

© Springer Nature Switzerland AG 2018
S. Monga and D. Benoit, *Assessing and Treating Anxiety Disorders in Young Children*, https://doi.org/10.1007/978-3-030-04939-3_12

in the daycare or classroom setting, the strategies they learn in the Taming Sneaky Fears program.
4. Highlight some of the points to keep in mind when parents and daycare and school professionals work with children who refuse to go to daycare or school.

12.2   Role of Daycare and School Professionals

Daycare providers, teachers, psychologists, social workers, speech and language clinicians, guidance counselors, and other school professionals play an important role in the management of childhood anxiety disorders, as these professionals can help young anxious children transfer and apply the skills they learn in the Taming Sneaky Fears program (and other mental health counseling programs) into the daycare or classroom setting. This is especially true with disorders such as separation anxiety disorder (characterized by children having difficulties separating from their parents, for example at drop off) and selective mutism and social anxiety disorder (characterized by children who do not speak and/or do not socialize). In daycare and school settings, the active involvement and participation of teachers and other daycare and school professionals can be key in the treatment process. Ideally, when daycare and school professionals work together with parents and clinicians to provide the necessary support to help young children generalize to the daycare or classroom the skills they learn in the Taming Sneaky Fears program, care is optimized. Additionally, daycare and school professionals could implement some of the basic strategies from the Taming Sneaky Fears program to enable young children who are shy and anxious, or those who worry excessively, to succeed in the classroom or as suggested in Sects. 6.2.2 and 6.2.3, the full program could be conducted in the daycare or school by school professionals.

12.2.1   Helping Parents Advocate for Their Children

When working with the parents of four- to seven-year-old children with an anxiety disorder, clinicians could encourage parents to seek out an understanding of how their child is behaving within the daycare or school; for example, within the classroom, at recess, and during other daycare- or school-related activities. Parents of young anxious children often indicate that they are not aware of what is transpiring at daycare or school between their children and peers, or between their children and the teachers.[4] In such situations, clinicians could inform parents that they can call and meet with the teacher or school administrators (and encourage them to do so) to obtain information about their children's performance and functioning and to advocate for

---

[4]From this point forward, 'teacher' refers to daycare providers and school professionals who work on a day-to-day basis with children.

resources and services. Occasionally, parents simply need to be provided with the information (and permission) to advocate for the appropriate resources in the daycare and school system for their children. In general, supporting parents as they advocate for the necessary supports can be a useful role for clinicians working with four- to seven-year-old children with anxiety disorders and their parents.

12.2.2 Engaging and Working with Teachers

When working with daycares and schools an important first goal is to ensure that teachers and school administrators have an understanding and awareness of how anxiety symptoms and/or anxiety disorders present in young children within the daycare and school setting. Some anxious children can be quiet, eager to please, and non-disruptive in daycare or classroom settings so they can easily 'fly under the radar' and their anxiety symptoms remain undetected. Clinicians can encourage parents to specifically review with their children's teachers the information provided on pages 5–8 of the Parent Manual[5] (which highlights the distinction between anxiety and anxiety disorders and describes the various types of anxiety disorders in young children). Such information could help teachers and school administrators appreciate the difference between normative anxiety symptoms and an anxiety disorder. Clinicians could also urge parents to communicate with teachers (and school administrators as needed) on a regular basis in order to monitor their children's progress and share with various daycare and school personnel any other information from the Parent Manual that they think would be relevant and helpful.

Although parents can often appropriately advocate for their children within the context of the daycare or school setting, occasionally, direct intervention from the clinicians with the teacher or school administrator is beneficial, especially, when despite parental effort, it has been difficult to have the necessary resources put in place to support the needs of young anxious children. In these circumstances, it can be beneficial for clinicians, after obtaining the appropriate parents' authorization, to contact teachers or school administrators and provide them with further information about anxiety disorders and the children's specific diagnosis or diagnoses, as well as engaging in a discussion about the children's needs. Ideally, such a discussion would take place in the presence of the parents and relevant daycare and/or school professionals. When clinicians have completed an assessment report, with permission from parents, the sharing of such an assessment note with the daycare or school professionals could be beneficial. However, it is also important to ensure that information within the assessment note that is deemed confidential by parents is not disclosed in such correspondence (providing the parents with a copy of the assessment report could be another way to ensure that parents release to the daycare or school only information they wish to be released, as they then would have full

[5]The Parent Manual is provided as one of the Supplementary Materials of Chap. 6.

control over what parts of the report to release). It might also be helpful, and more expedient for clinicians, to develop a form letter of sorts, which can provide teachers and school administrators with information about the definition and prevalence of anxiety disorders, the symptom manifestations of various anxiety disorders in young children, and some basic strategies to use with anxious children in the daycare or school settings.

12.3   Recognizing Anxiety Within Daycare and School Settings

Anxiety symptoms in young children can manifest in various ways in daycare and school settings. For example, some young children with anxiety disorders may simply be more shy and quiet than their same age peers, while others may freeze when put in the spotlight. Some children may be more reserved and hesitant than their non-anxious peers and this may manifest as reluctance to try new things or hesitancy to be the first, and refusal to participate in some activities. Some anxious children may be unable to make decisions (e.g., choose an activity to do or decide on what to draw), or may be unable or unwilling to engage in new activities. This hesitancy or caution may lead teachers to perceive these children as 'stubborn' rather than anxious, when, in fact, these behaviors are anxiety-driven. Some young anxious children may be perfectionistic, and need to make sure that everything they do is 'perfectly perfect,' and as a result are often afraid of making mistakes. This perfectionism within the classroom may manifest as a need to redo things, erase mistakes, crumple or rip work that is felt to be 'not good enough'. Perfectionism can also manifest as a refusal to try new things, especially when children who are perfectionistic believe they will not be able to do something perfectly the first time they try. Other young anxious children may be unable to use their voice to communicate with some or all adults and peers. This could lead teachers to perceive the children as 'stubborn' and 'choosing' not to speak when, in fact, the mutism is anxiety-driven. Some young anxious children may seek reassurance incessantly, complain of not feeling well and want the teacher to call their parents to be picked up from school and brought home. As a result, many of the above-described manifestations of anxiety can oftentimes be viewed (and therefore labeled) as a behavioral problem (rather than an anxiety symptom) within the context of the daycare or classroom.

Most young children do well with routine, structure, and predictability. This is especially true for young anxious children who typically do not like change and may have a more difficult day when there are unexpected disruptions or changes to the daily routine, for example, having a substitute teacher. Some young anxious children are so adverse to transitions and changes that they may protest strongly, display a behavioral or emotional outburst, and cry when teachers simply move from one activity to another, such as going from reading stories to having music time. Additionally, the sensitivity to criticism commonly seen in anxious children may be exhibited as a child quickly and easily breaking into tears for what the teacher may perceive as an insignificant trigger (or no reason), and may be perceived by the teacher as emotional dysregulation, sadness, or depression rather than anxiety.

12.4 General Strategies Within the Daycare or Classroom Setting

Teachers can utilize a variety of general strategies within the daycare or classroom setting when mild or moderate anxiety symptoms in young children are noted. Clinicians could propose teachers use the following strategies:

1. Encourage socialization with peers—it can be beneficial to develop a buddy system so that children who have difficulties speaking or socializing with peers are paired with other peers (while being mindful of not letting the buddy speak for the quiet child).
2. Spend one-on-one time with young anxious children—socially anxious and shy children need time to 'warm up' in order to feel comfortable and spending one-on-one time with socially anxious or shy children allows them to become more comfortable, resulting in a decrease in anxiety and what is often paralyzing inhibition.
3. Set the expectation for speech, for example, by using the mantra, 'Even shy children need to use their voice,' to encourage verbal interactions.
4. Do not let children be labeled 'non-talkers' and do not let other children talk for shy or mute children; if other children consistently speak for shy or mute children, supportively inform the speaking children that quiet children have a voice and need to use it.
5. Provide containment around excessive or generalized worries by setting aside (or scheduling) a 'worry time' at a specific time during the day such that there is no talking or thinking of worries outside of this time; if the children have worries outside of the 'worry time,' the children can be instructed to place the worry in a 'worry box' and keep the 'worry box' locked up until it is 'worry time' (as recommended by Huebner, 2006).
6. Utilize distraction—rather than allowing children to speak excessively about their worries; focus the children on to other topics of interest, e.g., distract them with a fun activity.[6]
7. Work with the parents (and/or the clinicians involved with the children) to build and implement Bravery Ladders to use within the classroom.

---

[6]These strategies do not apply to children who show anxiety in the context of exposure to domestic violence and other forms of maltreatment.

12.5   Explaining the Taming Sneaky Fears Program to Teachers

Clinicians working with parents of anxious four- to seven-year-old children could encourage parents to provide information to teachers about the Taming Sneaky Fears group CBT program. Parents could review pages 8 and 9 from the Parent Manual, with teachers in order to provide them with an overview of how traditional CBT overlaps with the Taming Sneaky Fears CBT program.

Although a full review of the Parent Manual would allow for a comprehensive understanding of the Taming Sneaky Fears group CBT program, teachers often prefer a more condensed summary of key concepts. As such, clinicians (or parents) could share the following summary of the seven key concepts from the Taming Sneak Fears group CBT program with teachers:

1. How to Be a Feeling Catcher: when children are Feeling Catchers they can look for and identify (or 'catch') feelings that they experience. By completing a Body Scan, children learn to identify the physical signs and clues that are associated with different feelings and therefore they are able to recognize the presence of specific feelings—e.g., when I smile I know that I am feeling happy.
2. How to Be the Boss of My Body: this concept helps children understand that when they experience a negative feeling (which makes their body feel bad), they can utilize one of three relaxation strategies, Spaghetti Arms and Toes (or progressive muscle relaxation), Balloon Breathing (or diaphragmatic breathing), or Imagery, to calm their body down and thus be in control or be the Boss of their Body. Teachers could learn the relaxation scripts (pages 21–23 of the Parent Manual) and use them with the children.
3. The Feeling Thermometer: this concept helps children to gauge the intensity of their feelings. Teachers could use the concept of a Feeling Thermometer with all of the children in the class to gauge feeling intensities, i.e., is the feeling at a low intensity (1 or 2 on the 10-point Feeling Thermometer), or at a moderate intensity (5 or 6 on the Feeling Thermometer), or at a high intensity (9 or 10 on the Feeling Thermometer). Teachers can remind or teach children that when their feeling intensity is at a 5 or higher on the Feeling Thermometer, they are too upset to think clearly and need to use the relaxation strategies to calm their body down.
4. Externalization of anxiety: this concept helps make the abstract concept of anxiety concrete and allows young anxious children to learn that they can exert control over their anxiety. In the Taming Sneaky Fears group CBT program, anxiety is externalized through the use of the story character 'Sneaky Fears,' which are two jackals that sneak scary and untrue thoughts into the brain of the main story character in the storybook section of *Taming Sneaky Fears—Leo the Lion's story of bravery & Inside Leo's den: The workbook* (Benoit & Monga, 2018a, b). Teachers could learn that the externalization of anxiety allows children to understand that anxiety (Sneaky Fears) is something external to them and therefore they can 'talk back' to or ignore Sneaky Fears if they wish to. When teachers

understand the concept of Sneaky Fears this allows teachers to ask children who appear anxious if their Sneaky Fears are bothering them.

5. The Tricks that Sneaky Fears play: this concept helps young anxious children understand that Sneaky Fears play Tricks on children by 'sneaking' inaccurate or unhelpful thoughts, also known as cognitive distortions, into their brain that cause anxiety. Teachers can learn that the many cognitive distortions are distilled into three Tricks: Not telling the Truth, Exaggerating, and Only Showing the Bad Things. With such information, teachers can encourage children to be Trick Catchers in order to 'catch' the Tricks that Sneaky Fears play and can support children to figure out Sneaky Fears' Tricks when they note anxiety in children.

6. How to Be the Boss of My Brain: this concept helps children learn that by using the Trick Stoppers (or cognitive strategies), they can Be the Boss of their Brain. Teachers can benefit from understanding that there are three Trick Stoppers to Tame Sneaky Fears: Ignore Sneaky Fears, Think Brave Thoughts, and Talk to an Adult. Teachers also benefit from understanding that the Taming Sneaky Fears program encourages young anxious children to seek out the support of teachers, coaches, and other important adults in the daycare or at school to help problem solve when they are feeling anxious and nervous in these settings.

7. How to Climb My Bravery Ladders: this concept helps children face and overcome specific fears and phobias. Teachers play an essential role in implementing Bravery Ladders within the daycare and/or school system thus helping young anxious children who might have incapacitating fears of being seen and heard speaking (selective mutism), excessive shyness (social anxiety), or separation anxiety from caregivers (as further detailed in Sects. 12.6–12.9).

12.6 Rationale for Bravery Ladders

Engagement of teachers and school administrators is key prior to implementing a Bravery Ladder within the daycare or school setting. Parents and clinicians could share the points discussed in Sect. 12.2.2 through to Sect. 12.5 with teachers as a first step. However, parents and clinicians may need to provide greater explanation and rationale to teachers and school professionals on Bravery Ladders and the importance of implementing Bravery Ladders in the school setting. Although a comprehensive review of pages 40 to 49 of the Parent Manual could provide such a rationale for the use of Bravery Ladders, parents and clinicians could also review the following as a way in which provide to teachers and school administrators with a succinct synopsis of what a Bravery Ladder is and what purpose it serves:

1. Describe a Bravery Ladder as a way in which to understand the technique of progressive desensitization or gradual exposure.

2. Explain progressive desensitization or gradual exposure as a technique that consists of taking small, manageable steps to reach a goal that would usually be unreachable without these smaller steps (much like ladders have small steps to help someone climb, one step at a time, to reach something that would otherwise be out of reach).

3. Provide examples of specific fears that can be tackled with Bravery Ladders, such as fear of making mistakes (perfectionism), fear of being away from a parent (separation anxiety), fear of being seen and heard speaking (selective mutism), fear of being in the spotlight, judged, or doing something embarrassing (social anxiety), fear of dogs (or other animals or insects), fear of the dark, fear of heights, etc.

12.7   Essential Ingredients for Success with Bravery Ladders

When clinicians (or parents) work with teachers, it is helpful to provide information about several key elements that are essential in building a Bravery Ladder, including the time commitment required in order to correctly implement a Bravery Ladder (Sect. 12.7.1), ensuring appropriate incentives are used (Sect. 12.7.2), and making sure to change only one element at a time (i.e., per step). Section 12.8 provides additional details for separation anxiety and Sect. 12.9 provides additional details for selective mutism and/or social anxiety disorder.

As teachers help young anxious children climb a Bravery Ladder at daycare or school, they encourage the young anxious children to use the relaxation strategies (Spaghetti Arms and Toes, Balloon Breathing, and Imagery) just as the children get ready to climb each step of their Bravery Ladder. Teachers also help young anxious children use the Feeling Thermometer to help children gauge the feeling intensity before and after using the relaxation strategies. As a result, parents and/or clinicians ensure that the points discussed in Sect. 12.5, and those described below, are communicated to teachers, and that teachers have a solid understanding of these concepts prior to implementing a Bravery Ladder.

The essential ingredients for teachers to be aware of when implementing a successful Bravery Ladder in the school setting (as described on page 40 in the Parent Manual) can be summarized as follows:

1. Daily exposure to the feared situation is ideal with at minimum, exposure at least four times per week.
2. Exposure of at least 20 minutes each time is best.
3. Ensure rewards/incentives are motivating, and used often.
4. Make sure to remind the children to use the Feeling Thermometer often (and as needed) to gauge how nervous or scared they feel.
5. Encourage children to use Spaghetti Arms and Toes, Balloon Breathing, and/or Imagery until their Feeling Thermometer is down to a 1 or 2 (to help the children climb each step successfully).
6. Use a warm, encouraging, calm, and firm (not punitive) approach that conveys to children that they are capable of climbing the step.
7. Praise children often for their efforts (and use the style of praising that is most appropriate for the children's temperamental style) in order to encourage them

to continue to climb the steps of their Bravery Ladder (reminding the children of what rewards they are working towards can be motivating).

8. Encourage children to climb an additional step of the Bravery Ladder if they are able to successfully climb the expected step and there is still time left in the 20-minute exposure (make sure to remind the children that they could earn additional points by climbing one more step on the Bravery Ladder).
9. Supportively push young children to face their fears and make expectations of the children's behavior clear and realistic.
10. Consistently praise and reward children for showing the expected brave behavior.

12.7.1 Time Commitment to Implement Bravery Ladders in the Daycare or School Setting

The importance of working on Bravery Ladders in the daycare and school settings cannot be overemphasized, especially for specific anxiety disorders such as separation anxiety disorder, selective mutism, and social anxiety disorder. Given that teachers have many children to teach and that implementation of a Bravery Ladder requires a significant (and regular) time commitment, it can often be difficult to implement Bravery Ladders in a daycare or school setting. However, when teachers are able to do so, Bravery Ladders can be valuable and successful. Therefore, parents and/or clinicians need to discuss with teachers ahead of time the significant time commitment required for daily exposures of at least 20 minutes each time, with at least four exposures per week (at a minimum). If a teacher cannot implement a Bravery Ladder because of time commitments or other reasons, finding an alternate daycare or school professional can be useful (e.g., teacher's assistant, vice-principal, librarian, etc.).

Given the required time commitment, implementation of a Bravery Ladder often is best planned for before the start of the school day, or during the lunch hour, or after the end of the school day (as long as the school day does not become excessively long). Typically, with the start of grade school, children may have a recess time, or may have a secondary teacher for physical education or music class and then these times might be opportunities to work with the primary teacher. Open communication between parents (or clinicians) and teachers could also generate other creative options.

12.7.2 Incentives for Implementing Bravery Ladders at Daycare or School

Establishing a reward or incentive system to motivate a child to want to climb the steps of the Bravery Ladder in the classroom is essential for the success of Bravery

Ladders. Parents (or clinicians) need to ensure that teachers understand that although using a Bravery Ladder is a means to help children overcome a specific fear, when teachers are working with children on a Bravery Ladder, they are asking children to face their biggest fears and that can be very overwhelming. Therefore, parents (or clinicians), in collaboration with the teachers, need to come up with an incentive system that is motivating enough for young anxious children to want to climb each step and face each feared situation head on.

Educating teachers on the use of Effective Praise as outlined in the Parent Manual (page 12) could be a first step in developing an incentive system that is rewarding for children. Additionally, parents could utilize and ask teachers to implement the two-point incentive system (described in more detail on page 42 of the Parent Manual) in which teachers assign one point (or check mark or sticker) for trying to climb the step and one additional point (or check mark or sticker) for climbing the step successfully. This strategy works well, especially when combined with the establishment of benchmarks, for example, providing increasingly more special or desirable rewards when the children reach ten points (or check marks or stickers) then 20, 30, 40, 50, or each time they reach a new benchmark. Help teachers appreciate that by using a two-point reward system at each step of the Bravery Ladder, children face a win-win situation as children get one point for at least trying to climb the step and one additional point for successfully climbing the step as expected.

A discussion between teachers and parents of how rewards will be implemented within the context of the daycare or school is also important. It is helpful for teachers to be aware that the most effective rewards often involve spending special times or participating in special activities, which could be established within the school. Alternatively, a point system for special time at home with the parent could be developed as long as a clear method is established to provide regular (daily) feedback and follow-through of implementation of rewards between teacher and parents. Effective rewards at school could include playing a game with a teacher, being the teacher's helper, choosing a story for the class to listen to. The actual rewards for each benchmark must also be discussed prior to starting the incentive system.

12.8   Working with Children with Separation Anxiety Disorder

Children with separation anxiety often have difficulties with daycare or school attendance, and drop off can be difficult for these children. Developing and implementing a Bravery Ladder in the daycare or school setting to address the separation anxiety symptoms displayed at drop off could be an ideal way to manage these symptoms. It can be beneficial to provide education to teachers about the importance of establishing a clear goal and a name for the Bravery Ladder, which in the case of children with separation difficulties could be something like, 'My Bravery Ladder for going with my teacher (without crying or clinging to mom) when mom leaves at drop off in the morning.' Teachers also benefit from education about the need to identify specific elements of a Bravery Ladder and the importance of only changing one element at time (i.e., per step). With separation anxiety, these elements could include: behavior that is expected from the child (going with my teacher without crying or clinging to mom), feared situation (when mom leaves at drop off), and setting (at school). The Parent Manual provides more details about the steps that could be used to build a Bravery Ladder for separation difficulties within the school or daycare setting.

Prior to implementation of a Bravery Ladder for difficulties with separation at school, it is necessary to ensure that there are no safety concerns around the children's reluctance to attend school; for example, teasing or bullying at school by another peer.

12.9   Working with Children with Selective Mutism and/or Social Anxiety Disorder

Selective mutism and or social anxiety disorder are exemplars for the need to implement a Bravery Ladder within a daycare or school setting, as young children with these anxiety disorders are typically able to speak and socialize easily and comfortably in the home and/or with some familiar adults, but their struggles arise primarily within the daycare or school setting. As such, there could be little need for implementation of a Bravery Ladder at home and instead the primary need for a Bravery Ladder is at daycare or school and specifically around speaking to a teacher (and/or socializing). Teachers generally benefit from understanding that all Bravery Ladders need to be implemented by an adult. Additionally, it is of value to help teachers understand and appreciate the importance of building a Bravery Ladder with a specific individual and the same individual (e.g., the same teacher or the same adult) through all steps of any specific Bravery Ladder. Explaining to teachers that in cases when there are several teachers to whom children do not speak and with whom they need to speak, then multiple Bravery Ladders (not all implemented at the same time) need to be developed, focusing on each teacher. It can be useful to re-emphasize to teachers that only one element of a Bravery Ladder can be changed at each step and therefore, if the volume of the child's voice is the element being changed on one step, no other element can be changed on that step.

As mentioned, teachers may benefit from being informed of the need to have a specific goal and hence a specific name for a Bravery Ladder. As described in the Parent Manual, an example of a Bravery Ladder for selective mutism could be 'My Bravery Ladder for using my normal voice to say five words to my teacher in the classroom.' Here, the four elements making up the Bravery Ladder are: (1) the voice volume (my normal voice), (2) the number of words (five words), (3) the person to whom the child will say the words (my teacher), and (4) the setting in which the child will say the words (in the classroom). Having such a detailed and specific Bravery Ladder title for selective mutism helps parents and teachers to more easily come up with the steps of the Bravery Ladder. The details on how to build a Bravery Ladder for selective mutism found in the Parent Manual (pages 42–47) could be discussed and shared with teachers in order to implement a Bravery Ladder in the daycare or school setting.

12.10   Conclusions

There can be immense benefits in developing a strong working relationship among parents, clinician(s), teachers, and school administrators to help manage the symptoms of anxiety in four- to seven-year-old children. Anxiety symptoms and anxiety disorders are prevalent among four- to seven-year-old children and yet they are very often missed within the daycare and school settings due to occasional lack of awareness of anxiety symptoms in young children, the often quiet nature of young anxious children, and the common mistaken interpretation of the anxiety as a behavior problem or as sadness/depression. When teachers and school administrators have an understanding of how anxiety symptoms present in young children, they have an opportunity to recognize and support these children early on. Early intervention from professional services in conjunction with strong collaborative support from teachers and school administrators could lead to more effective management of young children with anxiety disorders, which in turn, could lead to an improvement in the children's overall functioning in the daycare or school setting. This chapter strives to highlight the important role that teachers could play in the management of anxiety disorders in four- to seven-year-old children, especially with young children with selective mutism, social anxiety, and separation anxiety. Additionally, the chapter provides information on how the implementation of some (or all) of the evidence-based strategies of the Taming Sneaky Fears group CBT program within the daycare or school setting could provide further support to young anxious children and allow them to generalize the skills that they learn through treatment programs such as the Taming Sneaky Fears group CBT program.

References

1. Benoit, D., & Monga, S. (2018a). *Apprivoiser les Peurs-pas-fines—L'histoire de bravoure de Léo le lionceau & Dans la tanière de Léo: Le cahier de travail*. Victoria, British Columbia: FriesenPress.
2. Benoit, D., & Monga, S. (2018b). *Taming Sneaky Fears—Leo the Lion's story of bravery & Inside Leo's den: The workbook*. Victoria, British Columbia: FriesenPress.
3. Huebner, D. (2006). *What to do when you worry too much—A kid's guide to overcoming anxiety*. Washington, DC: Magination Press.

Chapter 13
Conclusions and Future Directions

13.1 Conclusions

Our knowledge and understanding of anxiety disorders in four- to seven-year-old children is still in its infancy. This creates a wealth of exciting opportunities for researchers and clinicians to work cooperatively in order to elucidate poorly understood or unexplored questions and challenge current knowledge to propel the field forward, while keeping in mind the ultimate goal of helping young anxious children and their families.

There is now general acceptance that young children can develop anxiety symptoms and anxiety disorders. However, as discussed in Chap. 1, despite the recognition that anxiety disorders in children are highly prevalent disorders, there is still limited information on comorbidity patterns, both within the various anxiety disorders and between anxiety and other non-anxiety disorders, especially with respect to young children. Additionally, there is much work still needed to elucidate the risk and protective factors involved in the development and perpetuation of anxiety disorders in young children. The field requires rigorous and methodologically sound studies to unravel the complex interplay among biological, environmental, and sociocultural factors.

Furthermore, as discussed in Chap. 2, there is a paucity of validated screening and assessment tools developed specifically for use in four- to seven-year old children. The efforts of our group (Chap. 3) and those of others (Chap. 2) will hopefully spearhead additional efforts to improve conceptual frameworks, develop universally accepted definitions of anxiety disorders in young children, create and validate screening and assessment tools to reliably evaluate anxiety disorders in young children using stringent research designs and methods. Given the significant interference in social, emotional, academic, and family functioning that anxiety disorders in young children creates, further work is needed in the area of early identification and accurate assessment of anxiety disorders in young children.

© Springer Nature Switzerland AG 2018
S. Monga and D. Benoit, *Assessing and Treating Anxiety Disorders in Young Children*, https://doi.org/10.1007/978-3-030-04939-3_13

Relatedly, several teams have worked hard at adapting existing treatment programs or creating new ones to help young anxious children (Chap. 4). These efforts have yielded mixed results. There continues to be a need for the development of evidence-based treatment programs that are developmentally appropriate, young-child-friendly, and are both efficacious and effective. In an attempt to develop such a program, our group created and refined the Taming Sneaky Fears group Cognitive Behavior Therapy (CBT) program for four- to seven-year-old anxious children and their parents. Chap. 5 reviews the various endeavors to create and refine the Taming Sneaky Fears program. Chaps. 6–11 provide step-by-step instructions on how to implement the Taming Sneaky Fears group CBT program. Through ongoing evaluative research, this program has challenged, and, in fact, shattered the long-held belief that children under age eight are too cognitively immature and unsophisticated to understand and process complex and abstract CBT concepts. Research with the Taming Sneaky Fears group CBT program has not only documented its efficacy in the treatment of preschool anxiety disorders, but also demonstrated that four- to seven-year-old children can learn complex and abstract CBT concepts when they are introduced in a developmentally appropriate manner. The Taming Sneaky Fears program is a valuable first step in the establishment of an evidence-based treatment of anxiety disorders in young children. We look forward to the Taming Sneaky Fears program being used by professionals from various disciplines and further evaluated by various research teams.

13.2 Future Directions

From a clinical perspective, we hope that the growing knowledge base about preschool anxiety disorders is widely disseminated among various health and mental health clinicians and primary care providers. Too often, preschool anxiety disorders are not recognized, or are dismissed and minimized. Although some symptoms of anxiety are normative, a sensitive, developmentally appropriate assessment is needed to ensure that anxiety disorders in young preschool children are not missed. This is particularly important given that many anxiety disorders in young children do not improve without treatment and significantly interfere with multiple areas of functioning. It is our hope that this book is a resource for clinicians as they work to help young four- to seven-year-old children learn age-appropriate coping strategies for managing their anxiety symptoms and overcoming their fears.

For the researcher, the field of anxiety disorders in young children offers many exciting avenues for exploration. All areas of preschool anxiety warrant thoughtful, methodologically sound research that carefully evaluates all aspects of preschool anxiety, including the determination of factors that contribute to the development and perpetuation of anxiety disorders (which could eventually lead to the prevention of these disorders), the development of validated, sensitive and specific screening and assessment tools to allow early detection of anxiety disorder (which would require universally accepted definitions and a more unified classification system for various anxiety disorders), and the further study of the efficacy and effectiveness of intervention programs for the treatment of young anxious children. We firmly believe that the best is yet to come.

Index

Printed by Printforce, the Netherlands